STANDARD
LOAN

UNLESS RECALLED BY ANOTHER READER
THIS ITEM MAY BE BORROWED FOR
FOUR WEEKS

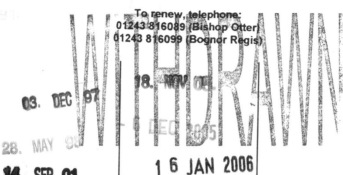

Multilingual Matters

Please contact us for the latest book information:
Multilingual Matters,
Bank House, 8a Hill Rd,
Clevedon, Avon BS21 7HH,
England

The Path to Language

Bilingual Education
for Deaf Children

Danielle Bouvet

Translated by Julie E. Johnson

MULTILINGUAL MATTERS LTD
Clevedon • Philadelphia

To all the deaf children I so deeply admire

*You who suffer at the hands of Science
because Science has remained deaf
to what it would learn from you*

Library of Congress Cataloging in Publication Data

Bouvet, Danielle
(Parole de l'enfant sourd. English)
The Path to Learning: Toward Bilingual Education for Deaf Children/Danielle
Bouvet, translated by Julie E. Johnson.
p. cm.
Translation of: La parole de l'enfant sourd.
Includes bibliographical references.
1. Children, Deaf — Language. 2. Deaf — Means of Communication. 3. Sign
Language — Study and Teaching. 4. Education, Bilingual. I. Title.
HV2391   1990
419   dc20

British Library Cataloguing in Publication Data

Bouvet, Danielle
The Path to Learning: Toward Bilingual Education for Deaf Children.
1. Deaf Children. Education.
I. Title. II. La parole de l'enfant sourd. *English.*
371.912

ISBN 1-85359-079-7
ISBN 1-85359-078-9 pbk

Multilingual Matters Ltd

Bank House, 8a Hill Road   &   1900 Frost Road, Suite 101
Clevedon, Avon BS21 7HH   Bristol, PA 19007
England   U.S.A.

Copyright © 1990 Danielle Bouvet.
Translated by Julie E. Johnson.

First published in 1982 under the title 'La parole de l'enfant sourd' by Presses
Universitaires de France, Paris, France.

Typeset by Editorial Enterprises, Torquay, Devon.
Printed and bound in Great Britain by WBC Print Ltd.

Contents

Preface

In *For a Child to Speak*, Danielle Bouvet presents the findings of her research and her fascinating work with deaf children. In conjunction with a congenitally deaf counterpart, she offers a bilingual class in which deaf children learn and communicate in both Sign Language and oral language. While the children are shown how to communicate with hearing people through lipreading and using their voice, they are also grounded in Sign Language — a language which affords them the ability to construct innumerable statements and which contributes to their psychical development.

In Bouvet's classroom, it would be out of the question to forbid these deaf children to express themselves with gestures, as was done in the past, and force them to use oral language. This interdiction never kept the deaf from using gestures among themselves anyway. But it did make traditional rehabilitation a particularly laborious process which relied upon training drills that condemned the children to systematic frustrations many were unable to endure. In a bilingual class, the hearing teacher often finds herself just as handicapped in the face of Sign Language as the deaf children do in the face of oral language. A bilingual class thus implicitly acknowledges the children's right to become who they really are.

Bouvet's work offers much more than practical methods of deaf education. Beginning with her own classroom experiences with deaf children, she inquires into the conditions of child language development in general, and reevaluates the connection between language acquisition and cognitive development. Her findings are important for all those who work in child psychology and child psychiatry.

Educating or rehabilitating a congenitally deaf child is not a simple matter even though the techniques generally applied have been used for many years. Suzanne Borel-Maisonny, under whom Bouvet studied, significantly advanced rehabilitation techniques by perfecting ingenious ways to help deaf children become aware of internal voice-related movements and vibrations and to connect these perceived forms to phonemes. Yet for all the infinite patience, firm authority, and monotony-breaking creativity this exacting work demands, one question remains. How can one teach a child who is handicapped, and thus at a clear disadvantage, what other children normally never have to be taught?

Language development was long considered, explicitly and implicitly, as something to be taken for granted. It was assumed to happen naturally as the body grew and the organs developed. Of course, given the plurality of languages, scholars admitted that cultural environment must play some role. But until the eighteenth century, they still pondered which fundamental language a child would speak if removed at birth from those speaking the local language (would it be Greek, Latin, Hebrew?). While such questions eventually ceased to be a subject of debate, a naive, unexpressed hypothesis continued to underlie many approaches to rehabilitation. Namely, since linguistic communication was an innate property of man, removing a few barriers or supplying the constituent elements of speech was all that was necessary in order for language to develop. Handicapped children would then eagerly use it as if this bit of help was all they had needed. (Apparently, deaf children lacked these elements of speech only by chance, as the result of an illness or a congenital anomaly.)

Observations of the deaf have long shown that deaf children's desire for communication quickly brings them to use a more direct and less difficult mode among themselves. Under such conditions it is not easy to convince them to use oral language for their own pleasure.

Children do not learn to speak unless they are immersed in a world where others speak. Nor can adults 'teach' a child to speak in the narrow sense of the word. Nonetheless, this is precisely what special educators working with deaf children — and speech therapists working with dysphasic and sensorially handicapped children — are still often asked to do. For their efforts to have meaning, they must take into account the conditions under which langauge develops. This is far more important than analyzing what a child without language lacks. Moreover, there is a danger that such analyses could create a fundamental disorder where none existed, the disorder being but the reflection of the system against which the child's deficiency was analyzed.

All children, whether destined to be hearing or deaf, are conceived, carried, and brought into the world by parents who live in a world of language. In that world, children find their place, their name, and their fantasy-life well before they come into sensory contact with their parents' language. While children without any sensory handicap who belong to likewise unimpaired parents enjoy the most advantages, deaf children of deaf parents are, from the first days of life, better off than deaf children of hearing parents.

The first rudiments of communication appear very early. From the first weeks of life, children specifically react to the faces around them, which are composed of elements that engage all the senses of sight, hearing (the voice of the mother or mother-figure immediately plays an important role), smell, and kinesthesia, in which tonal dialogue is important (J. de Ajuriaguerra). At this initial stage, the absence of one of the senses probably does not radically modify the development of these elementary precursors to communication. The mother does not know that her child is deaf and continues to talk to him or her just as to a hearing child. A few-months-old infant is literally immersed in language. Only a very depressed mother or a nurse obsessed with the fear of contaminating the infants in her charge will care for a baby in silence. How curious and playful is the language of adults talking to a baby. Each one knows that the infant doesn't understand what is said to him or her, yet all speak with the greatest sincerity.

As children change and develop psychically, they acquire this purposeless speech, addressed to no one in particular, and mix it in with their own language games.

For children living under average conditions, language rapidly grows richer in vocabulary and syntactic structures toward the end of the second year. At that point children clearly begin appropriating statements that have been made to them, and become capable of transforming these statements to fit their own purposes. Meanwhile, they start appropriating what they have heard people say around, but not to them. Growing up means identifying with parents and other adults and what one imagines they are like when not interacting with children — a process that involves talking as grown-ups do when they think children can't hear them. This is how swear words get introduced into even the most puritan of families. It is in living with adults and with children who already speak that a child acquires the mother tongue which all use but no one teaches.

For deaf children, a break unfortunately occurs at a critical moment in psychical development. When, under usual conditions, a baby begins to babble, very particular exchanges develop between the infant and those around it. Babblings, we have long known, tend to reproduce the general melody of adult language. To explain this phenomenon, we must recognize that pleasurable proprioception necessarily integrates into the child's schema, the origins of which are undeniably sensory in nature and linked to auditory stimuli. Such stimuli are precisely what deaf children lack. More recently, another integrative tendency, symmetrical to the first, has also gained recognition. Namely, adults in turn adapt the intonations of their speech to match the melody of a baby's babblings. Such echoing games surely bring infants as much pleasure as exchanging smiles, which they generally begin enjoying much earlier.

Such melodic dialogues never develop with a deaf infant. An attentive mother immediately notices this, even if she hasn't yet pinpointed just what is missing. At that moment, a deaf child's development begins to diverge from the norm and become marked by the child's inability to pick up speech—whether addressed to him or not—and by the mother's dismay. She feels stifled when interacting with her baby, sensing that what, for her, gives meaning to things and to emotions is missing.

With the diagnosis made, all the problems associated with intervening specialists begin to arise. Traditionally, specialists tried to console parents who were traumatized by the news that their child was deaf by promising to make their child speak. From that point on, everything that had allowed the child non-oral modes of communication was considered a hinderance to the treatment that might eliminate the original infliction. Non-hearing children were thus deprived of all allowable forms of communication. Meanwhile, those around them wondered why some children became agitated, depressed, or rebellious against efforts to make them speak orally.

For a deaf counselor to teach parents the 'signed' mother tongue early on, the parents obviously have to accept the fact that their child is deaf right away. But such acceptance spares them from having to experience a breakdown in communication that can have heavy consequences for them and their child. For deaf parents acceptance comes a lot easier; they know that, like themselves, their deaf child is a complete person.

Later intervention efforts must take into account the various registers of language used by ordinary children — particularly language for play — once they can experience themselves as separate from their mother. The language of gestures is the only language deaf children can play with among themselves. Thus, a school for these children must not be organized according to the traditional model, defined by individual or group rehabilitation classes and rooms. School must first and foremost be a place of life — a place where the children, along with each other and their teachers, can experience what deafness keeps them from experiencing elsewhere. Isn't this what school should be for all children unable to enjoy these fundamental experiences of play at home?

In Danielle Bouvet's bilingual class, the children get to see their two teachers talking with each other. One is deaf, the other hearing. And each respects the other's way of life. As a team they tell fun stories that the children enjoy together with their teachers.

I encourage all those who care for children struggling with oral and written language to read this book. It will stimulate their thinking far beyond the issues of deaf children.

René Diatkine

Introduction

Speech is what defines the human child. The word *infant*, composed of *in* (not) and *fari* (speak), means 'doesn't speak'.

We thus perceive infants in terms of something they lack, something they are missing. Yet we sense that this lack will be a temporary, passing phase and go so far as to give these little 'speechless' beings a name even before they are born. And from the moment of birth we treat them as subjects who will be able to talk and call themselves by name.

Although they do not yet talk, we welcome them as *speaking subjects*, as if our very confidence will bring forth the speech we so eagerly anticipate. In fact, so strong is our expectation, that speech acquisition is assumed to be a natural development, the result of a biological process directly linked to the maturation of the nervous system. We do not doubt that one day these little-ones will walk and talk. But walking and talking are two quite different processes. Walking is indeed essentially a function of how the human body naturally develops; but talking, or speech acquisition, is a highly socialized process intimately connected with children's first interactions with those around them.

We might feel that both walking and talking develop naturally, almost regardless of outside factors. But we must admit that there is a difference when it comes to remembering these two accomplishments: those close to a child remember quite clearly when he or she took those famous *first steps*, but are hard pressed to place the child's *first words*.

How can we possibly pin-point just when an event as expected and anticipated as speech actually occurred?

Those first words are the 'greatest gift' any child can give, yet they seem to elude us, lost in the blur between expectation and reality. What makes this 'greatest gift' so difficult to place in time is the fact that it is offered within an on-going relationship of interpersonal exchange. Without such a relationship speech cannot emerge.

Conventional wisdom often throws walking and talking together, but the advent of speech and the development of ambulatory skills are two entirely different phenomena. Attesting to this is the fact that children all follow a similar pattern when beginning to walk, but vary widely in learning to talk.

In a paper entitled 'A psychiatric approach to dysphasia', Réné Diatkine (1975b) notes that in a large population of four year-old schoolchildren, one third spoke with great ease and made themselves understood remarkably well, another third were much less clear in their speech, and the last third were unable to make themselves understood through speech alone. These differences are due to multiple factors connected to socio-cultural and socio-economic conditions. As Diatkine affirms, a child's early psychic make-up, 'which is linked to his first relationships, his first desires and his first fears' (Diatkine, 1975a: 12) greatly influences how he will acquire speech.

Such early differences in speech ability are at the root of numerous scholastic failures as early as the first grade, for schooling is based on the assumption that children have already mastered basic verbal communication skills before the first day of class. Yet the fact is that only a minority of first-graders have attained this level of verbal competence, namely those who come from a healthy language-learning environment.

The preconceived notion that language develops almost spontaneously and can be taken for granted clearly penalizes many hearing children. For deaf children, the consequences of this assumption are even more devastating. Babies who are born deaf are *infants* too: tiny human beings whom we perceive as speechless, and whose speech we fully anticipate. Deaf children thus enter the world as *speaking subjects* and are welcomed as ordinary children. The fact that they don't hear the sounds of speech may go unnoticed for a long time, for even though words cannot reach them, they are perfectly able to use their voice. In their first three months, deaf children's lallations are just like those of other children's. These kinesthetically-based vocalizations result from the activity of voice organs — organs which are intact in deaf children.

One can well imagine then how dramatically the diagnosis of deafness can change the way in which we relate to a child: instead of looking forward to the infant's speech we lament the prospect of his or her muteness. Historically, deaf children have long been labelled as 'deaf-mutes'. Even today many people still subconsciously associate deafness with muteness. Those close to a deaf baby thus struggle against immense confusion, for there is no way to reconcile the notion of *muteness* with that of the *infant* (who *will* speak). In the process of being diagnosed, deaf children can lose their status as *infants* — lose their status as speaking subjects. In sum, the *diagnosis of deafness* makes them appear to be *paradoxical subjects.*

Yet muteness is in no way correlated to deafness.

It is deaf children who suffer most from our ill-founded assumption that speech is acquired automatically, regardless of one's learning environment. Such assumptions can be harmful to hearing children, but they do even greater damage to deaf children: by insisting on speech that we take for granted, we plunge deaf children into greater paradox, for we refuse to perceive them but in terms of the one thing they lack.

People tend to think about the ability or inability to speak in absolute terms. Yet as the following pages will show, things are not so black and white.

In Part One we take a fresh look at how speech functions and how children acquire it. This provides the theoretical basis for Part Two, in which we observe that there are many more similarities than differences between deaf and hearing children — even when it comes to speech. Upon this theoretical foundation we established a pilot program involving six deaf children — five profoundly deaf and one severely deaf. A description and the results of this undertaking are presented in Part Three.

The purpose of the present work is to define the situation of deaf children — not merely in terms of what they lack, but in terms of what they really live. In taking this dual theoretical/clinical approach, we come to see that deaf children are full-fledged speaking subjects just like hearing children.

Our conclusions offer new insights into how we all might more appropriately respond to deaf children as speaking beings and thus better meet their educational needs.

Part One:
Acquiring Speech

We cannot understand the language abilities and needs of deaf children unless we possess an in-depth knowledge of how ordinary children acquire speech. To acquire language, a deaf child must benefit from the same learning conditions as any hearing child.

Accordingly, the aim of Part One is to identify those conditions. To do so, however, we must closely examine speech itself. What are we really doing when we speak? How do children acquire speech? What do we really mean by 'mother tongue'? Our first three chapters are devoted to answering these questions, for they form the very basis of our approach to deaf children.

Children learn to speak by playing with words.
René Diatkine

1 What are We Doing When We Speak?

When we speak, when we communicate through language, we do so with sentences, not isolated words. Even if these sentences are truncated or incomplete, they are sentences nonetheless. True, some statements can be reduced to a single word, but only because they are part of a verbal exchange and have a precise place in a precise linguistic context. A sentence doesn't just exist; it must be created by a speaking subject. It is the result of a speaker actualizing certain semantic possibilities of a sign system in order to say something. As such, a sentence is not merely the sum of the signs that constitute it; its essence lies at a different level.

So that we can better understand what it is we are doing when we speak, we will first study the nature of the linguistic sign and then attempt to define the place of the speaking subject in the speech process

The Nature of the Linguistic Sign[1] and its Occurrence in the Speech Process

In a paper entitled 'Form and Meaning in Language', Emile Benveniste (1974: 235) distinguishes 'between the language units called *signs*, considered in themselves and as meaning something, and the *statement*[2] where the same elements are constructed and juxtaposed to make a particular utterance'. This distinction leads to two different approaches to linguistics.

The first linguistic approach, which began with Ferdinand de Saussure, studies the sign as a signifying element, but does not study or define what it signifies. The sign is intra-linguistic or *semiotic*; it exists to the extent that it is part of a network, defined in relation and in opposition to other signs within the language. In terms of the semiotic sign, 'to be distinctive and significant are one and the same' (Benveniste, 1974: 223). During a discussion with Benveniste, the French philosopher Paul Ricoeur once pointed out that this linguistic approach creates the following paradox: 'The sign disappears in its essential function, which is to say something' (ibid.: 236).

The second linguistic approach, introduced by Benveniste, starts with the semiotic, the closed world of signs, and leads 'to things beyond language' (ibid.: 225). This is a *semantic* approach, based not on the sign but on the statement. As Benveniste puts it: 'The semiotic is characterized as a property of language; the semantic results from an activity of the speaker who puts language into action' (ibid.: 225).

These two linguistic philosophies — language as *semiotic* or *semantic* — provide two separate definitions of meaning in language. From the *semiotic* perspective, meaning is defined in terms of other signs and does not refer back to particular things. Meaning is not established in relation to the referent. In the *semantic* view, on the other hand, the statement occurs in 'the realm of language in use and in action' (ibid.: 224), and relates to what is real. Only the particular has meaning; meaning is 'what the speaker intends to say, the linguistic actualization of his thought' (ibid.: 225). The meaning of the word — the basic semantic sign — can be defined only in terms of its syntagmatic relationship to the rest of the statement: 'The meaning of a word is its use' (ibid.: 226), that is, the way it reflects back to a referent.

Because of this semiotic/semantic duality in linguistics, any one linguistic element may be seen either semiotically or semantically — as a *sign* or as a *word*. Semiotic signs belong to the treasure chest of available signs. They are 'conceptual, generic, non-circumstantial'. Words, on the other hand, are the instruments of semantic expression. They translate 'notions which are always particular, specific, and circumstantial through accepted contingent uses of speech' (ibid.: 228).

Although the semiotic sign is fundamental to language, it is not everything. Language is more than a system for signifying, for it is also the meeting place of semantic activity. Language serves as a 'mediator between one man and another, between man and the world' (ibid.: 224). The semiotic sign is a significant unit that carries meaning, yet its meaning depends on the context in which it occurs. Which brings us back to the semantic, for the occurrences, or *tokens*, of the semiotic sign are what constitute the semantic sign. We will now take a closer look at how the semantic sign functions.

The semantic sign or 'the sign considered also as a thing'

The semantic sign or 'word' retains only part of its value as a semiotic sign — it is a *thing* that represents another thing. This is somewhat similar to the way the sign was viewed in classical philosophy. The diagram $x \rightarrow y$ (x representing the sign and y the thing represented) shows the paradox that French and Anglo-Saxon philosophers came up against from the seventeenth century to the nineteenth century. The paradox can be presented as follows: the sign must be transparent in order to lead to the thing represented, yet the thing represented cannot be reached without the presence of the sign. Thus the sign must not be totally transparent — otherwise it cannot be seen. It must maintain a certain opaqueness in order to exist also as a *thing*.

François Récanati (1979a) explains the paradox of the sign being both transparent and opaque as follows:

> Considered as a *thing*, the sign focuses the 'mind's eye' on itself. It is the very object of consideration. It doesn't 'represent' anything; rather it presents itself ($\overset{\frown}{x}$). As a *sign*, however, it escapes consideration and shifts the mind's eye from itself to the object that it signifies ($x \rightarrow y$). The sign is like a mirror that reflects something other than itself, or again like a transparent windowpane that permits a view of something beyond itself. Yet both the mirror and the windowpane have the property of becoming opaque; that is, they can shed their transparency and instead offer themselves for consideration, present themselves to the mind's eye. An object can cease being considered as a *sign* and be considered as a *thing*. As a result it ceases to be linked to the thing signified and recovers its independence as a *thing*; the object no longer shifts attention away from itself, but instead presents itself for consideration. It becomes opaque and loses the transparency that made it possible to see the second object through it. (Récanati 1979a: 33)

It was the resolution of this paradox that led to the theory of consciousness, to the Cartesian 'I think', according to which thought reflects back on itself at the same time that it represents its object. Representativity is thus connected to reflexivity in that what is thought cannot be separated from the fact of thinking it. This means that the sign is no longer regarded only in its transparency or only in its opaqueness, but in a third state of 'transparency-cum-opaqueness'. 'The sign, neither transparent ($x \rightarrow y$), nor opaque ($\overset{\frown}{x}$), is both transparent and opaque ($\overset{\frown}{x} \rightarrow y$)', suggests Récanati. 'It reflects back on itself at the same time that it represents something other than itself' (ibid.: 21).

Récanati notes that these problems, which concerned philosophers in the classical age, do not seem to exercise many contemporary thinkers. In this day and age, when everything seems to be viewed in psychological terms, philosophers cling to an inherited mode of reasoning that radically separates the *fact of thinking* from *what is thought*.

And yet a few scholars such as Wittgenstein (in his later works), Austin and Strawson — all of whom study ordinary language from the perspective of analytical philosophy — have truly returned to the classical tradition of the sign. Their studies of actual utterances have placed anew an emphasis on the reflexivity of language. These scholars argue against the notion of a fully transparent language ($x{\rightarrow}y$) which values only the representative function of language and ignores its pragmatic dimension, namely, its use in discourse.

Like the sign, the utterance speaks both of the thing it represents and of itself; that is, it goes on representing, though reflected (and reflected upon) as a fact in itself. The utterance thus simultaneously performs a representative and a metalinguistic function; it represents something else while presenting itself. Even when an expression is put in quotation marks, which makes it somewhat opaque, its transparency and representativity continue to function effectively.

Let us take the example given by Récanati: '*Monsieur Auguste*' *est venu* ('Monsieur Auguste' came by) (1979a: 78–79). In this utterance, the single quotation marks indicate an exaggerated intonation meant to highlight the deference and even the servility of the expression 'Monsieur August' as it was used by another speaker. Although the expression 'Monsieur Auguste' is offset and presented with a certain amount of metalinguistic distance as an object of speech, it still clearly represents the person referred to as well. The expression 'Monsieur Auguste' represents Auguste while reflecting on its own materiality. It is thus symbolized by the diagram ($\overset{\frown}{x}{\rightarrow}y$). 'The sign does not vanish as a *thing* itself in the face of what it represents', concludes Récanati (ibid.: 87).

This notion of the semantic sign will be the key to our approach throughout this work. Now let us consider the implications of this notion when applied to the act of speaking.

Speaking is both saying and showing: token-reflexivity

Benveniste and Austin independently discovered the special nature of certain expressions such as 'I congratulate you'. Rather than describe or represent a prior and independent fact, these words constitute the very fact that resides in the utterance 'I congratulate you'. Taking another example, Benveniste (1971: 229) writes: 'The utterance "I swear" is the very act which pledges me, not the description of the act that I am performing... The utterance is identified with the act itself'.

Austin calls such expressions 'performative'. An utterance is said to be performative, explains Oswald Ducrot (1972: 69), 'if it satisfies two conditions: (1)

interpreted literally, it describes a concurrent action of the speaker; (2) the specific function of the utterance is to perform this action'. Thus, by saying 'I promise', 'I do what I say I am doing by the simple fact that I say I am doing it' (ibid.: 69). This would not hold true for utterances such as 'I am talking' or 'I am taking a walk', which might be called *constative* since they do not create a new reality, but simply describe a preexisting one.

In performative utterances, there is no duality between the representor and the represented. Such utterances are 'are "*sui*-referential" in that they reflexively indicate the type of act that their enunciation accomplishes' (Récanati 1979a: 107). Thus performative utterances actually accomplish the act they refer to and can be represented as $(\overset{\frown}{x})$ (as opposed to the constative $(x{\rightarrow}y)$).

It was through the above type of unusual expressions that Austin discovered performativity. He then realized that the concept could, by extension, apply to all utterances since any utterance can be paraphrased to include an explicit performative. 'I am taking a walk', for example, can be paraphrased as 'I state that I am taking a walk', and to say 'I state' is to *perform the act of stating something*. In other words, 'I state' is an explicit performative. 'I am taking a walk' can thus be considered a primary performative utterance. This means that the presumed distinction between what would be called performative and constative utterances actually does not exist.

Austin thus destroyed the illusion of purely constative utterances. He also refutes the idea that an utterance can be purely performative, reduced merely to a speech act. Every utterance presents a *locutionary* aspect (what is said, the content) and an *illocutionary* aspect (the speech act itself, be it an affirmation, a question, a promise, or whatever). While referring to a state of things $(x{\rightarrow}y)$, the utterance reflects back on itself as an act $(\overset{\frown}{x})$. Thus the diagram previously introduced, $\overset{\frown}{x}{\rightarrow}y$, is the one that fully accounts for every utterance.

By showing that language is always performative we have also shown that it is always reflexive. We can hence discard the notion that language is a purely representative activity that precludes, *ipso facto*, any trace of reflexivity.

In addition to being fully compatible with representation as a function of language, reflexivity is also consistent with monstration, or what language shows. In Wittgenstein's view, not everything can be said through language, but what can't be said can be expressed by being shown. In other words, that which we cannot express (say) *through* language can be expressed (shown) *in* language. Récanati (1979a) explains this double aspect of language as follows:

> Language does more than represent; it also shows, and what it shows is precisely that which it cannot represent. Reflexivity, set apart from representation, is an accepted aspect of monstration. The representor shows itself,

exhibiting its formal properties at the same time that it represents the represented. (Récanati, 1979a: 126)

Every utterance, in other words, describes or represents a fact — this is
what is *said*. Every utterance is also an act, an act of making an affirmation, pos-
ing a question, etc. — this is what is *shown*. An affirmative utterance *shows* that
it is an affirmation, it does not describe itself as such.

Every utterance thus functions in two ways: it reflects (or shows) itself and
it also represents (or says) something beyond itself. The utterance is both a *thing*
and a *sign*. Every utterance presents itself as *thing* while continuing to function
as a *sign* that refers to what is said.

Thus, according to philosophers who study ordinary language and who recognize the dual nature of the classical sign as both a *thing* and a *sign*, speaking
is indeed both saying and showing.

Before Austin, linguists such as Bally, Jespersen, Jakobson and Benveniste
had observed the distinctive nature of certain expressions such as 'I', 'you',
'this' and 'now'. These expressions seem to be singular examples of the above
discussion. They function as indexical symbols that *show*, like a pointing finger.
An index pointed in the direction of an apple designates that apple. So does saying 'this apple', if the speaker is right near it. Or take the words 'I' and 'you'.
Unless we are given the context in which they are said, we can't tell who the referents are. This is because such expressions identify their referents in terms of
the *de facto* relationship between their *token* (their occurrence in speech) and the
objects they designate. Each token of the expression corresponds to a different
referent, and that referent cannot be identified unless we consider the token in
the precise context of a particular utterance.

Hans Reichenbach calls such expressions 'token-reflexive'. 'The opacifica-
tion of these expressions is a *sine qua non* condition of their transparency... in
order to represent things, they present themselves as *things*', explains Récanati
(1979a: 163). As an *utterance-type*, token-reflexive expressions have only general significance. But when they are used in a particular utterance, the token
lends them specific meaning, which in turn designates their specific referents.

An example will clarify these distinctions: If x says, 'I am tired', x is the
referent of the token 'I'. We know what 'I' means and to whom it refers because
the token presents the referent as the one pronouncing the statement 'I am tired'.

Like the phenomenon of performativity, the phenomenon of token-reflexivity is not limited to the singular expressions that led to its discovery. It can
be extended to utterances containing these expressions. The meaning of the
utterance

involves that utterance's reference to itself, just as the meaning of the token-reflexive expression within it involves the expression's self-reference. Consequently, an utterance containing a token-reflexive expression is itself token reflexive: the token-reflexivity is transmitted from the words to the utterances. (Récanati, 1979a: 162)

Moreover, certain authors maintain that every means we use to talk about particular objects resorts to token-reflexivity, whether this means be a definite description (a noun accompanied by a definite article), a proper name, a demonstrative, an indexical symbol or a determiner.

For example, the utterance 'the cat is on the mat' refers back to a particular cat and a particular mat if and only if we take into account the singular event of its being uttered, that is, its token. The fact of the utterance is certainly reflected in the meaning of the statement, and through this meaning we can determine the reference.

The relationship between words and what is being talked about through them is mediated by the intentional use of those words by speaking subjects: depending upon the person speaking and the situation, the expression 'the cat' will designate such and such a cat'. (Récanati, 1979a: 50)

Obviously, we cannot disregard this pragmatic dimension of language, namely, the impact of discourse on language.

To understand an utterance is not only to know what it signifies as a sentence-type at a semiotic level. One must also be able to grasp its actual meaning through the token-reflexivity of referential expressions. However, none of this can happen unless the hearer is able to ascertain what to make of the utterance as a speech act. This is very clear in detective novel dialogues. The meaning of certain statements escapes the reader's understanding unless the utterance reveals how it should be taken — as a threat, an order, etc. In Récanati's (1979a: 174) words, 'Reference is possible only in the larger context of an illocutionary act'. Just as statements are not true speech acts unless they reflect back on themselves, illocutionary acts cannot be performed without being token-reflexive.

Hence, the utterance reflects itself twice over, first in the token-reflexivity of its referential expressions, and secondly in its token-reflexivity as an illocutionary act. Now let us further explore the illocutionary act itself.

Speaking is also making a calculation

An illocutionary act is not complete until it is effectively understood by the hearer. This is what Austin means when he uses the word *uptake*. Uptake is not accomplished simply by making an intentional speech act — this intention must be recognized by the hearer.

> This unique property of discursive communication means that the intention of S (the speaker) is not a simple intention of communicating to H (the hearer) a content *p*, but a complex and reflexive intention of communicating *p* to H by means of H recognizing this intention. (Récanati, 1979b: 95)

Performative verbs are a sure means to this end. 'They ensure the hearer's recognition of the speaker's illocutionary intention by shedding full light on his intention and ruling out the possibility of this intention going unrecognized' (ibid.: 180).

Intentional implication (*sous-entendu*) is another sure way of making one's intentions understood. Before considering the processes involved in intentional implication we must first present the conversational rules established by Paul Grice (1975) in his article, 'Logic and Conversation'. Grice describes the regular behaviors that appear in any process of linguistic communication and that derive from a general principle which he calls 'the principle of cooperation'. This principle leads to rules of conversation, which he classifies in four categories:

(i) *Quantity*

- Make your contribution as informative as is required for the current purposes of the exchange.
- Do not make your contribution more informative than is required (this point is also covered by the rule of relevance).

(ii) *Quality*

- Try to make your contribution one that is true:
(a) do not say what you believe to be false
(b) do not say that for which you lack adequate evidence

(iii) *Relation*

- Be relevant. Grice (1975: 47) emphasizes that 'though the maxim itself is terse, its formulation conceals a number of problems that exercise me a good deal'.

(iv) *Manner*

- Be perspicuous:
(a) avoid obscurity of expression;
(b) avoid ambiguity;

(c) be brief;

(d) be orderly, etc.

Even though (as Grice recognizes) these rules are not of equal importance, they all enter into the calculation of conversational implication in the same way. Some authors, such as Dan Sperber (1974) and François Flahault (1978), argue that these rules can even be reduced to a single principle: *relevance*.

We assume that when people speak, they are respecting the rules of speech. This is what Récanati (1979a, 188) calls 'Presumed Respect of the Rules' (PRR): 'To reconcile the presumed respect of the rules by all speakers and the particular contribution of a specific speaker, the hearer is led to make certain hypotheses' (ibid.: 190). Thus when I say, 'the cat is on the mat', I *give to understand* that I am respecting the rule of quality. The hearer can hypothesize that I in fact believe that the cat is on the mat. Grice calls this kind of hypothesis 'trivial'. Trivial hypotheses constitute the *pragmatic implications* of the utterance.

In referring to non-trivial hypotheses that are not a direct application of PRR, Grice speaks of 'conversational implication'. This could be a situation in which a speaker allows a certain premise to be understood from his utterance. For example, if a speaker tells a driver whose car has broken down that there is a garage at the next light, the driver may hypothesize that this utterance implies that the garage is very likely to be open, for he believes that to speak of a closed garage would be incompatible with the Presumed Respect of the Rules. It must be pointed out, however, that although the hearer might hypothesize that the garage is open, the speaker has done nothing to ensure that the hearer recognizes this hypothesis. He has merely *allowed* the implication of his utterance to be understood, that is all.

Récanati has identified other situations in which the speaker actually alerts the hearer to the fact that he intends to lead him to make a specific hypothesis. This is no longer to *allow* something to be understood but to *intentionally imply it*. Here the speaker truly performs an indirect speech act with guaranteed uptake. Récanati (1979b) explains:

> In order to have an intentional implication there must be an outright violation of the rules and moreover, this violation must be unexplainable[3] except by the speaker meaning to intentionally imply something. The speaker's seemingly inexplicable violation of the principles of conversation is a signal that these principles are being respected at some level other than literal communication. Such a violation of the rules of conversation indicates that the speaker is purposely implying something and that his intent is 'disguised'. The infraction thus serves to shift gears from literal communication to implicit communication. (Récanati, 1979b: 104)

To illustrate this definition, we will take the example given by Alan H. Gardiner (1932: 231): 'Have you lost something?' As an illocutionary act the utterance poses a question. Yet taken in a precise context, it could be understood not as a question but as a very pointed request that the hearer leave.

How is this indirect speech act accomplished? When a speaker says to someone who is there loafing about in front of him, 'Have you lost something?' he is making an abnormal utterance which *for no apparent reason* violates the rule of relevance. The utterance does not fit the situation — the hearer clearly is not looking for anything at all. This open violation of a conversational rule alerts the hearer to the fact that the *true* message lies on a different plane. The hearer must thus reconstruct the implied premise in order to establish a conversation in which the rules will be respected. He could reason: 'The speaker is asking me this odd question because in order to remain standing here, one must have a good reason, such as looking for something he has lost. Since I don't have any such reason, I must leave'. By *intentional implication*, the speaker has clearly indicated to the hearer that he should leave. The speaker did not simply *allow* this request to be understood but *intentionally implied it* through an indirect speech act.

So not everything is said for the same purpose. Speech lends itself to implicit as well as explicit statements. Through implication we can say implicitly what, for any number of reasons, we don't wish to say explicitly. We use implication for the sake of courtesy, as in the above example, but also for many other reasons — to avoid being contradicted, for instance. This point is brought up by Ducrot (1972):

> A second possible origin of the need to be implicit has to do with the fact that any explicit affirmation automatically becomes a possible topic of discussion. Anything that is stated may be countered... Thus, if we are going to express a basic belief, be it relative to a social or personal issue, we resort to a means of expression that does not put it on display, does not make it an assignable object which may be contested. (Ducrot, 1972: 6)

To speak implicitly is to make an involved calculation about an utterance and about how it relates to the rules of conversation. The speaker makes this calculation openly and objectively to guarantee uptake of his 'indirect' speech act, that is, to ensure that his 'openly disguised' intentions are recognized (Récanati, 1979b: 99).

To understand this calculation the hearer must think about what could have prompted the speaker to say what he said. Here again, the act of enunciation must be taken into consideration in order to fully grasp the meaning of the statement.

In sum, speaking is also making a calculation that takes into account the very fact of the utterance, the reasons behind it and what it shows. In conversational implication we once again find the distinction between what is said, what is shown and what may be implied. On the one hand, intentional implication has to do with 'what is shown through speaking without really being part of what is said' (Récanati, 1979a: 211). On the other hand trivial, pragmatic implication and conversational implication that doesn't inexplicably violate the rules of conversation both belong to what may be implied.

Interpreting an utterance is more of a 'calculation' than it is a simple decoding exercise. Comprehension requires the active participation of a subject capable of making suppositions: speaking is also knowing how to make hypotheses.

Summary and presentation of a speech act observed in a deaf child

These few reflections on the nature of the linguistic sign were meant to show that, contrary to the conventional concept of language still widely accepted by educators of deaf children, language is not a transparent code that reflects directly back to what is said. Language emerges as a complex dialectic between saying and showing, between transparency and opaqueness. Only in this dialectic can we grasp the meaning of utterances: *what is said* cannot be understood without taking into account *the fact that it is said*.

Representation is not all there is to language: an utterance signifies by 'presenting itself' as much as it does by 'representing'. Like the linguistic sign, a word is both a *thing* and a *sign*. As a *thing*, it accomplishes a speech act and is opaque — illocutionary acts do not represent, they show. As a *sign*, however, a word represents something else and is therefore transparent.

The meaning of a word or utterance cannot be conveyed but through the synthesis of these two aspects. Only by recognizing this paradox can we begin to truly understand the speech process, which is very complex. If we overemphasize the phenomenon of representation, we lose sight of the reflexivity involved in monstration.

As we have seen, this reflexivity is always at work in explicit or implicit illocutionary acts, in referential expressions, and in the semantic sign — which, as a *thing*, 'does not vanish in the face of that which it represents' (Récanati, 1979a: 87).

The following real-life example illustrates how essential it is that we acknowledge these linguistic principles. It concerns a speech act observed in a nine-year-old child profoundly deaf from birth.

This child lives with his hearing family. Ever since his deafness was discovered when he was about two years old he has undergone regular speech therapy sessions. His deafness is such that he cannot spontaneously acquire any speech at all, even with a hearing aid.

One sunny afternoon in early spring we exchanged a few words as school let out. Both of us were delighted to see that Spring had finally come; in fact I myself was eager to get out and enjoy the weather. 'It's nice out... What are you going to do after school?' I asked. Since we often talked about his backyard, I expected him to answer that he would go out to play, to ride his bicycle or to be in the sun... But after making me ask the question several times so that he could read it on my lips, he answered, 'I am going to walk on the sidewalk...'. It took him some time to formulate this answer as he visibly summoned up all the effort and determination the response required. Needless to say, the performance was totally devoid of any pleasure!

The response left me deeply perplexed and raised a series of new questions in my mind in addition to all the uncertainties of a difficult profession ('making' the deaf talk). In fact, it was this response that prompted me to undertake extensive research and numerous endeavors, including the writing of this book.

Yes, the boy had answered me, but was his response an answer to my question or was it just a 'French' exercise performed 'in a vacuum' — something that had nothing to do with speech? I was speaking to him, but was he speaking to me? His sentence was perfectly structured syntactically: 'I am going to walk on the sidewalk'. But was it an utterance? Was this the utterance of a speaking subject participating in a conversation? In context, the sentence was a complete *non sequitur* not even remotely relevant to the situation at hand. It didn't seem like an utterance at all because no speaking subject was apparent — the sentence didn't seem to belong to anyone. The child had answered me without any uptake of my question; that is, he did not recognize my intention of asking him how he planned to spend that particular afternoon, the very first afternoon of Spring. Yet my question would have been clear to any child who can hear.

The boy had answered only the question 'do what?'. He knows that this type of question is answered with a verb. But he didn't make any calculation to determine how my question was to be taken. He related to his own enunciation as though it were merely a *statement*, not something *he* was saying.

As we have seen, no statement can be interpreted independently from the act of enunciation. So it is hardly surprising that this child was unable to grasp the meaning of my question.

Talking with this child was not easy. He 'spoke' willingly in grammar or vocabulary 'exercises'. But when he was addressed directly with a view to communication, he often appeared disconcerted and even shocked: why would someone want to ask *him* a question? I tried to explain to him that I liked him and was interested in what he did outside school. I tried to tell him that we talk to each other because it is enjoyable. But I knew how futile it was to say such things to a child who had never had the opportunity to discover them on his own.

Even though he was somewhat familiar with the linguistic code used around him, this child was obviously unaware of rules of usage, for he hadn't the least idea *what people are doing when they speak.*

Although he 'spoke', he didn't know what it meant to converse and thus didn't see any point in it. His answer was an answer to *a* question, but not to *my* question because he didn't understand my utterance as an act.

In the context of our exchange, the child's answer is a 'statement' that says nothing. It is drained of any real content because it relates exclusively to what was said and not to its being said. He produced a statement that would never have been made by a hearing subject in the same utterance situation; for a hearing subject uses the code knowing the rules about how it is applied in speech. But the deaf child, unaware of conversational rules, is unfamiliar with the rule of relevance — you don't state the obvious (such as walking on the sidewalk) when someone asks you a question in the hope of obtaining interesting information.

This speech act brings to mind a situation presented by Flahault in his book *La Parole Intermédiaire* (1978). Flahault imagines what would happen if a sign saying 'Please stay off the grass' were posted in a subway station. The traveler could not take it but

> as an utterance which, though perfectly intelligible linguistically, is absurd in the situation and has no value as a meaningful notice that 'someone' posted. The request would be devoid of any value as an utterance and thus also devoid of any illocutionary bearing. But it would indeed make the traveler wonder, 'Who in the world put that up?' (Flahault, 1978: 112)

Here, the speaking subject is unrecognizable because the statement is irrelevant to the situation in which it is presented. If, however, this same statement were found posted in the middle of a lawn in a public park, the passerby would take it as a perfectly appropriate utterance and naturally attribute it to 'someone' with the authority to make such a request.

In order to have an utterance (i. e. in order for a statement to be 'owned' by a speaking subject) what is said must be pertinent and appropriate to the situation; otherwise no speaking subject can be identified.

This explains what happened in the conversation between the deaf child and myself. The tragedy is that in this case we are no longer in the realm of an imagined situation, but are speaking of a widespread reality.

Even after years working with deaf children, one can't help but be struck when they make statements like this which don't really say anything in the context of the conversation, statements which a hearing child would never produce in the same situation. Yet in and of themselves these utterances say a lot about the incoherent way in which we 'make' deaf children talk, basing our approach on an utterly erroneous philosophy that reduces the speech process to simply knowing a code. No instruction aimed at merely teaching a code will ever help children understand the speech process. Indeed, 'it would be, as we say, "impossible" to talk with someone who seemed incapable of anything more than producing syntactically correct statements or who understood only what was "literally" stated' (Flahault, 1979: 75).

I certainly couldn't talk with this deaf child, this 'de-muted' child capable of producing sentences and using a code but incapable of speaking and conversing. Had we not destroyed *his* speech? Had we not deeply wounded him as a speaking subject — all in the name of de-muting him? This is the theme we will now explore by considering the speaking subject's place in the speech process.

The Speaking Subject's Place in the Speech Process

Words are spoken to be heard. They create or presuppose a relationship between the two or more people who are talking with each other. Even when we 'talk to ourselves' there is a relationship involved, namely, our relationship with ourselves, as indicated by the reflexive pronoun. Yet soliloquy is not considered to be a fully normal use of speech, for speech fundamentally implies that there is someone being spoken to. The inherent purpose of verbal activity is to connect with others.

Verbal relationships are characterized by the unique manner in which they occur: the interlocutors share a specific segment of time, *speech time*. In verbal activity, the one talking and the one (or those) listening always *take turns*. We can talk only one at a time. According to Flahault (1979: 74), 'this adherence of several people to a single thread of time — which replaces the different and parallel time continuums lived by each before entering into the speech relationship' — constitutes or establishes the very possibility of a speech process at all.

Even before 'taking' his or her turn speaking, each interlocutor is already suspended or tied to this single thread of speech time and engaged in a relative relationship to it. Because this space in time is shared, it imposes a strategy on the interlocutors.

Speech-space is not 'neutral ground': it implies a tactical approach. This fact is evident in everyday expressions such as 'take the floor', 'get a word in edgewise', 'cut someone off', etc.

Such expressions highlight the fact that there are two aspects to the speech process which must be taken into consideration: the *process* inherent to the exchange, and the *content* or information to be transmitted, that is, what is said.

Too often we forget that a piece of information (the *content*) cannot be transmitted unless a whole series of phenomena (the *process*) occurs between the interlocutors.

These two aspects of speech are also found in the various accepted definitions of the verb 'to communicate'. In the expression 'to communicate something to someone', the verb means 'to transmit a piece of information'. But it can also mean 'to be in relationship', as in the expression 'these two rooms communicate'. This meaning found in the intransitive construction seems to have been the first accepted definition of the Latin verb *communicare*, meaning 'to be in relationship with'.

We can't understand what linguistic communication is all about unless we consider both of these aspects: the transmission of content, and the process of making contact which makes this transmission possible (Lepot-Froment, 1979: 18).

Many people think of linguistic communication only in terms of content and completely disregard the primary and fundamental process of 'entering into relationship'. If, on the contrary, we define linguistic communication in terms of the process, then the content, still accounted for, emerges as 'a way of "entering into relationship" with others' (Flahault, 1978: 25). This concept of language not only accounts for both *content* and *process*, but places them in a hierarchy relative to each other.

Why are these two aspects kept so separate in the traditional concept of language? According to Flahault (1978),

> the answer clearly lies in the tendency to differentiate between the subject as a being and his attribute as "speaking". This distinction necessarily means that language can be considered only as an instrument, used essentially to transmit information. (Flahault, 1978: 25)

In this view, speech is the emblem of a preexisting person.

Benveniste was the first linguist to disagree with this instrumentalist concept of language, which had been generally accepted as 'obvious'. Realizing what a stir his approach might cause, he prefaces his assertions with the observation that 'it is sometimes useful to require proof of the obvious' (Benveniste, 1971: 253). In Benveniste's (1971) view, this likening of language to an instrument or invention is completely unjustified:

> Language is in the nature of man, and he did not fabricate it. We are always inclined to that naive concept of a primordial period in which a complete man discovered another one, equally complete, and between the two of them language was worked out little by little. This is pure fiction. We can never get back to man separated from language and we shall never see him inventing it... It is a speaking man whom we find in the world, a man speaking to another man, and language provides the very definition of man' (ibid.: 224).

By accounting for the existence of 'man in language', Benveniste opened up a new line of linguistic research. In terms of this new approach, we can go so far as to say that the person or subject can come to exist only in and through language. The only subject is a 'speaking subject'.

Here we get back to what was presented in the introduction to the present work: infants enter the world as speaking subjects with their own given name. They are subjects whom we address, to whom we speak. Our intuitions tell us that there can be no such thing as a speechless subject. This is what goes unacknowledged in the instrumentalist concept of language.

How then do subjects come to exist through the speech process itself? This is what we will now consider.

Speaking is becoming a subject

Along the path from birth to their first words, children go through a complex process that transforms their pure subjectivity into relative objectivity, and in this objectivity they begin to discover the real world as they discover themselves and come to exist as subjects.

The way children go through this process is by interacting in a relationship and by speaking.

Human young are born with great dependency on maternal care; without it they could not survive. In responding almost perfectly to all of their infant's needs, mothers allow their child to live in a state of fusion. Oblivious to any separation between 'inner reality' and 'outer reality', infants remain unaware of their many limitations and know only a feeling of omnipotence. Though good and necessary, maternal adaptation to the needs of a newborn baby leaves no room for interaction between mother and child as two separate individuals.

But very early on mothers begin to lessen their nearly total adaptation, and the process of separation begins. Separation allows children to 'benefit' from the experience of want, which will make them aware of their limitations. They can then begin to discover themselves while also discovering 'the other'. As children and their mother thus emerge as two individuals they enter into an interactive relationship.

The theory of psychoanalysis has brought to light the important role that expectation and the emergence of desire play in a child's self-discovery. In his theory of primary maternal preoccupation, D. W. Winnicott (1971) explains the process as follows:

> The good-enough mother... starts off with an almost complete adaptation to her infant's needs, and as time proceeds she adapts less and less completely, gradually, according to the infant's growing ability to deal with her failure... *If all goes well*, the infant can actually come to gain from the experience of frustration, since incomplete adaptation to need makes objects real, that is to say, hated as well as loved. The fact is, *if all goes well*, prolonged close adaptation to need that isn't allowed its natural decrease can actually disturb the child because exact adaptation resembles magic and the object that behaves perfectly becomes no better than a hallucination. (Winnicott, 1971: 10–11)

Only through want and gradual frustration can children discover the objectivity of the outside world and correspondingly experience their own existence.

Yet any frustration, as gradual and necessary as it may be, leads to strong feelings of anxiety in children as they become 'disillusioned' with their feelings of omnipotence and experience the chasm of want and absence. In order to focus this anxiety and make it bearable, children take up all sorts of 'transitional' activities that allow them to face the separation between their inner world and the outer world.

It was Winnicott who identified the transitional tactics children use to deal with their anxiety when the contrast between presence and absence would otherwise be too great to bear. He observed that at a point of separation — before going to sleep, for example — children will seek out a specific object or engage in a particular activity (suck their thumb, rock back and forth, murmur) as a way of fighting against the anxiety of separation. In this way the children put themselves in a 'transitional' space that, according to Winnicott, allows them to avoid the problem of inside versus outside, of Me versus not-Me.

Parents intuitively recognize the stress their children experience at these moments of separation and are careful to give them an object that calms them. Depending on the child, this might be a teddy bear, a diaper, or what have you, but it will always be the same one. Children shift their attachment to this 'transitional' object which, for them, evokes their mother's presence.

Although this tactic has obvious advantages, in the long run it may fail. Diatkine (1973) has noted the problems it can cause and how children deal with them:

> A wooden bobbin is not a mother and too much confusion between them might lead to a situation as undesirable as the one at the outset. This is why another system of separation and opposition develops at the same time so the child can quickly and perfectly differentiate between them while attributing a sort of comparable affective value to each. This is the point at which language enters in and *denomination* plays an extremely important role. (Diatkine, 1973: 137).

Through language and naming, children discover the possibility of better regulating their pleasure-displeasure system by better controlling the anxiety of separation.

Through denomination, children lend the 'named' object an affective value comparable to that of their mother's presence. This creates *distinction* rather than *confusion* between the object and the mother's presence. Herein lies the advantage of denomination over the transitional object. The only way children can transfer their attachment to a transitional object is by confusing the Me and the not-Me. Yet in the end, the transitional object cannot match the expected pleasure and by its very nature it 'quickly loses that which at the beginning made it special' (Diatkine, 1976: 603).

Once children become capable of internalizing their mother by placing her within themselves, they can face separation and come to exist as subjects relative to this other person whose distinct existence they are discovering. There is no 'I' without a 'you', and this differentiation is what leads to an awareness of objective reality.

This is where language comes into play. The fact that children name and distinguish things shows that they are able to represent and deal with absence. But in order to face separation, children need to have experienced continuity in their first relationships — they have to have known presence. This is why it takes longer for language to develop in children who have experienced too much upheaval in their early relationships.

Children's beginning to name things, however, does not mean that they won't continue to keep a large part of their psychical activity in the blur of the transitional space — a space in which they do not have to come to terms with the contrast between inside and outside. Although subjects come to exist in and through speech, this does not happen overnight in an 'all or nothing' process. Quite to the contrary, it is a matter of continual development: as human beings we never stop discovering reality and coming to exist as subjects.

We make this quest in one very special way, namely, through speech. As Jacques Lacan (1977: 40) reminds us, this is unequivocally so in psychoanalysis, which 'has only a single medium: the patient's speech'. The feeling for one's own existence emerges from an awareness of the existence of another person. Through this distinction we discover objective reality and realize that relationships always involve some third element, that they are not dual but triangular: 'No subject can establish himself alone and outside of language (not even with another person if this duo does not reflect off a distinct third element that situates each in relation to the other)' (Flahault, 1978: 161).

In sum, speech can originate only in an atmosphere of communication and interaction, and can bring the subject into existence only by weaving him or her into an entire web of human relationships. This is the process we will now further examine.

Speaking is also 'finding one's place'

Every time we speak we inevitably assume and/or are put in a particular place. How is this so?

As Benveniste points out, the pronouns 'I' and 'you' function in complex ways in speech. The word 'I', he explains, is not merely an economical way of naming oneself, it is a term that I use to refer to myself only when I am addressing someone who will also use this term to refer to himself when he speaks to me. The term 'I' is thus inconceivable without the term 'you', which again we will both use to designate each other as we speak. The two terms are

complementary, although according to an 'interior/exterior' opposition, and at the same time, they are reversible. If we seek a parallel to this, we will not find it. The condition of man in language is unique. (Benveniste, 1971: 225)

We would have to disagree — there does exist a parallel to this linguistic process, namely the identification process by which children begin to develop an inside/outside distinction between themselves and their mother. At first this distinction can develop only in a state of reversibility — it is to the extent that children can interiorize their mother that they are able to emerge as subjects and recognize their mother as a partner having a distinct existence.

This striking parallel between linguistic process and psychical development further justifies a linguistic approach which accounts for the existence of 'man in language' (Benveniste, 1971: 193). 'Man' and 'language' are not two distinct realities — they are inseparable. The one cannot exist without the other.

In the same vein as ordinary-language philosophers and as Ducrot, Flahault (1978: 70) shows that the impact of speech reaches far beyond the illocutionary act to affect the very existence of the subjects: 'All speech, even the most harmless of small-talk, involves illocution; and illocution resides in "who you are for me and who I am for you"'. Insofar as statements are concerned, speech is a matter of *cognition*, but at a much more fundamental level, speech is a matter of human relationship, that is, *recognition*.

Illocutionary acts always involve an act of recognition between the people who are speaking to each other, an act which assigns a place to each of them. 'Speech is always produced from a certain place and always calls upon the interlocutor to assume a corresponding one', explains Flahault (1978: 58).

This same notion of language comes through in the following passage by Lacan (1973):

> We have always distinguished two levels on which humans converse. First there is recognition. Speech creates a bond between the subjects which transforms and establishes them as humans involved in communication. Then there is what is communicated. Here we distinguish all sorts of sublevels: summoning, discussing, knowing, informing. (Lacan, 1973: 125).

Speaking, then, is a process which 'establishes' people in a bond of recognition from which they each draw their sense of existence. After recognizing that speech has the unique quality of bringing subjects to exist, Flahault developed the concept of 'subject realization space'. This is the space where the subjects find themselves caught in a whole network of constraints and limitations. It is a space where they 'always find illusions, injustices, and a disconcerting abundance of that's-just-the-way-it-is predicaments' (Flahault, 1978: 154). Such give and take assigns a role to each person. As in the work place, each person has a function to serve. Flahault makes it clear that he means 'role' in this sense and not as role-playing or taking on a character. In his view, no 'free-thinker' can claim that his or her individuality remains unaffected by the role he or she is assigned within the speech process itself.

Clearly, the subject realization space is not neutral but full of violence. Though it does not involve physical violence, it does require the speakers to engage in a 'positioning' process in which they each must establish their respective place; for if this relationship is not defined, speech is not possible.

Flahault offers us a very revealing example on this subject. During an adult training seminar, each participant was to present a subject of his or her choice to the group. A man named Alexander announced that he was going to talk about hunting wild boar. At first he came over as sounding like a textbook. He was uneasy and so were his listeners. Then he drew a diagram on the blackboard to show how the hunters were arranged and pointed out where he himself had been positioned, saying, 'I was here'. From that moment on his presentation came alive and his audience was enthralled. What happened? Flahault (1978) explains that at first,

> Alexander was trying to assume the position of someone who has his facts straight. The rules of the game entitled him to his turn, but as someone in middle management and of working class origins, he didn't feel qualified to take the floor except on the merits of Knowledge — the kind of knowledge claimed by authoritative speakers who back up what they say with books. Since this position inspired respect in Alexander, he thought that it would impress others. But in this situation, all it did was impede his ability to speak. The place where he got back on his feet was where he 'became himself again' so to speak. (Flahault, 1978: 69)

Influenced as he was by his schooling and upbringing, Alexander had been unable to express himself because he felt impelled to speak from someone else's position, namely that of the 'authoritative' speaker. Here we see that the subject realization space can violate the subject in the process of assigning places, for the subject ends up 'talking the way he imagines he is heard' (Barthes, 1978: 10).

According to Flahault, speakers do enjoy a certain degree of freedom in that they do not preexist language but establish themselves as they speak. Yet there are limits to this freedom, for it takes wing from a place where roles are assigned, where speech 'always subjectively includes its own reply' (Lacan, 1977: 85). Flahault rejects the myth that speech is a creative process in which the subject is utterly free to take advantage of any and all of the multiple ways language can be shuffled and rearranged, for this myth does not take into account the act of recognition involved in any verbal interaction.

Flahault's concept of the subject realization space also accounts for our extensive and varied use of speech that 'says nothing' — that endless flow of rather uninformative words that spill from our mouths throughout the day. This is one verbal phenomenon that language theories based essentially on the transmission of information have never been able to explain adequately.

To account for such speech in all its varied forms, from 'Hello, do you hear me?' at the beginning of a phone conversation, to 'profuse exchanges of ritualized formulas', Jakobson (1960: 355) resorts to the notion of a 'phatic function', which he defines as 'a set for CONTACT'. But saying 'Hello, do you hear me?' to make sure that you have a good connection and have made 'contact' at physical level, is not the same as exchanging ritualized formulas for which the physical contact has already been established. The phatic function fails to explain the use of these formulas.

In fact, the whole notion of a phatic function is highly questionable. It is presented as a function of contact *outside* of what is said. Yet we have already established that the process of 'entering into relationship' is essential to, and cannot be separated from, what is said, that is, the content, which in itself draws us into relationship with others.

Since ritualized expressions make up such an important part of all verbal interaction, a theory of language should be able to account for them as part of verbal activity in general, and not have to treat them separately as marginal or secondary.

The exchange of ritualized formulas is perfectly explainable when we consider that speech takes place in a process of recognition. These formulas may not offer much in the way of *cognition*, but they lead to *recognition* on the level of human relationship. After they have been uttered, each person is slightly different, both to him or herself and to the other. In this light, these formulas can be seen as a way of approaching each other and defining each person's place so that a dialogue can ensue. But just like any other type of speech, ritualized formulas can also be a way for the interlocutors to 'maintain or uphold a sense of their own existence through achieving an exchange' (Flahault, 1978: 158). This exchange may not reflect any content, but it is an exchange nonetheless.

As Flahault conceptualizes them, these ritualized formulas thus arise from a normal use of speech. And this fact constitutes a further argument in favor of the approach we have been supporting. According to this approach, the essential properties of speech include such fundamentals as establishing the existence of the speakers and affording them the means to affirm themselves in their own and each other's eyes.

For those who have found themselves in a foreign country where they didn't know the language, this theoretical approach rings all too true! We experience painful feelings of non-existence when such circumstances temporarily deprive us of speech and the ability to situate ourselves in verbal interaction.

Similarly, we all know that people who live alone 'without anyone whom [they can] really talk to' (Saint-Exupéry, 1946: 8) will often carry on long conversations with a pet as a way of keeping their feelings of non-existence at bay. To a certain extent, this is also why people talk to themselves.

We have seen how our sense of existence is tied to the speech process and anchored in a web of human relationships. These relationships are established as we speak with each other, one subject to another according to the diagram($S \leftrightarrows S$). But in a physical sense, speech also reflects back on itself. The diagram thus becomes ($\widehat{S} \leftrightarrows \widehat{S}$). Let us focus now on this physical aspect of speech.

Speaking is hearing, expressing and identifying oneself

Here we come back to the notion of reflexivity that we previously examined in relation to the linguistic sign. We have seen that the sign has value not only because it is transparent, but also because it is opaque and constitutes a *thing*. Now, from the speaker's perspective, we discover that the sign's materiality is important for another reason: signs cannot be physically produced except in reflexivity, namely the reflexivity which occurs between the motor and sensory mechanisms involved in speech. As we speak, our speech-producing motor activities are constantly being monitored by our sense of sound so that we can continually adjust our articulatory movements. In other words, every articulation of the voice reflects back on itself through the sense of sound. We wouldn't be able to speak if it weren't for this unique aural monitoring circuit and the feedback it continually shoots back and forth between what we hear and how we articulate.

Speaking thus requires that one's hearing be intact, not only to know what others are saying, but also to be able to regulate one's own voice production. This internal feedback constitutes one of the main characteristics of all linguistic communication and is the phenomenon that makes speech reflexive even as a physical reality. Let us examine this phenomenon more closely.

Babies do not wait until they can speak to produce sounds. Right from birth they readily make all sorts of sounds that serve various functions. They can make sounds to express well-being or suffering. They also make sounds for the sheer pleasure of the way it feels cenesthetically or kinesthetically in their diaphragm, lungs, larynx, palate, tongue, teeth and lips when they restrain or release a column of air. Furthermore, making sounds gives babies the chance to experiment with their aural perceptions and to develop that fine-tuned synergy between voice articulation and its corresponding sound images. Babies develop a coordination between what they hear and how they use their voice by playing with sounds — and how delighted they are when they discover their abilities! Ruth Weir (1966) observed that even at six months, babies raised in an environment where Chinese (a tonal language) is spoken, produce utterly different sounds from babies raised in a French-speaking environment. Similarly, Philip Lieberman (1967) showed that the voice pitch of babies raised essentially by their father is different from that of babies raised by their mother.

As we can see, the sounds that babies hear around them influence their babbling from a very early age, for babbling essentially emerges from the aural-articulatory circuit. Babbling is far from being speech, but it already exhibits one of the main characteristics of speech: self-regulation through hearing. Little by little, a child's babbling conforms to repeating the sounds that he or she hears.

We tend to think of spoken words as 'fleeting' compared to the permanence of written words. But actually quite the opposite is true: spoken words begin settling deep inside each of us in our tender infancy, molding our ear and the sounds we make long before we ever speak.

When it comes to the sounds of language, children produce what they hear. In essence, another person's speech comes to inhabit them. First and foremost, this other person is their mother — they drink in her sounds as they drink in her milk. The very materiality of language becomes a source of pleasure for infants when they find that they can recreate something of the presence of their mother and identify with her by producing sounds.

This brings us back to the process by which speaking subjects establish themselves. There is no 'I' without an internalized 'you'. In like fashion, infants must receive another person's speech before they can produce their own.

Even when children have acquired their first words and can 'have their say', they still enjoy playing with signifiers. A good part of their speech is reserved exclusively for their favorite game: playing with sounds. We have seen that the linguistic sign is an opaque *thing* as well as a transparent *sign*. Children demonstrate this in the way that they play with words — it doesn't really matter what the words mean, they're just fun *things* to juggle and fit together for their rhythm and rhyme.

This enjoyment does not disappear with childhood. The lure and appeal of sounds are evident in the way we use language day in and day out. Jakobson (1960: 356) discusses this appeal in his article 'Linguistics and Poetics'. The poetic function, he asserts, is not limited to poetry alone. To one degree or another it affects all language. Any verbal activity is poetic in that it reveals the 'palpability of signs'.

In a sequence of two coordinate names that are not affected by any hierarchy, we tend to start with the shortest one in order to give the message a 'well-ordered shape' (ibid.: 357). We also like to pair off similar-sounding words. We'd sooner say 'Horrible Harry' than 'dreadful', 'terrible', 'frightful' or 'disgusting' Harry (ibid.: 357). Without realizing it, we fall back on the poetic device of juxtaposing similar sounds. Advertisers are well aware that the better an advertising slogan sounds, the better its 'ring', the greater its impact will be on the target audience.

In his article, 'About the Sound Mm...', Ralph Greenson (1954: 235–236) shows that mere vocal qualities can charge even an isolated sound with meaning. Take, for example, the sound 'Mm...' made in a long murmur. Greenson suggests that this sound evokes the pleasure of food, which relates back to a baby's pleasure of nursing at his or her mother's breast. The sound is produced, and can be prolonged, by holding the lips together as one would to not let go of something held in the mouth. Greenson notes that this 'Mm...' sound, which carries rich and satisfying connotations linked to nursing, is often used in advertisements for desserts, soups and other dishes or foods to convey how delicious they are. Not surprisingly, we find this sound in the word meaning 'mother' in many languages: 'mère' in French, 'mutter' in German, 'madre' in Spanish and Italian, 'meter' in Greek, 'mater' in Latin, 'ama' in Albanian, 'ummu' in Assyrian and 'em' in Hebrew (Greenson, 1954: 235-236).

Because speech always depends upon the aural-articulatory circuit and requires that subjects be able to hear themselves, even the sounds of speech become charged with meaning. In fact, much of our language activity is inspired by the way a message sounds. Here again subjects find themselves 'caught' in a web — the web of sound related emotions and meaning that signifiers, echoing from their earliest experiences and attachments in life, might evoke.

Yet the physical aspect of sounds offers the subject a place of relatively free spontaneous expression and inner release. Here, each of us can reestablish 'old liberties and get rid of the burden of intellectual upbringing' (Freud, 1960: 127). We can break the subjugation of speech produced within the constraints of a positioning process.

To hear oneself is to discover a personal expression of who we are in the world of signifiers. Here we mean 'expression' in its etymological sense: the hearing-regulated expulsion of air that becomes our speech and 'posits' us as it vibrates in the glottis and resonates in all of our various vocal cavities. Expression is not a matter of 'receiving' a place but of 'taking' one. In fact, sometimes we end up expressing more than we intend. Our true emotions and sentiments are sometimes betrayed by the way our words actually come out sounding!

To hear oneself is also to form an identity, insofar as our own speech resembles that of people around us. Socio-linguistic research has shown that different ways of speaking and articulating can be a strong factor in social cohesion. We recognize ourselves as speakers belonging to a particular group.

In sum, speech is not the least bit 'innocent', even in a physical sense. Since we can never escape the sound of our own voice, speech reflects everything we each have lived. In fact, our sensitivity to certain sounds can dredge up what lies in our deepest self.

There is always a physical dimension to speech. Sometimes this dimension is even featured, as in poetry, songs and plays on words. But speech can never escape vocal effects altogether: speaking always involves playing-playing with the sound matter of speech.

Summary and what speaking is for a deaf person

In the preceding discussion on the place of the speaker in the speech process, we contested the instrumentalist view of language which presents the subject as preexisting and 'detached' from that process, language being a tool that came later, a tool that we fashioned in order to communicate with other individuals. We attempted to show that, quite to the contrary, speech forms the subject and vice versa. It is in and through language that each subject emerges into his or her own existence. *There is no subject but a speaking subject.* To refute this dimension of language by considering language a mere instrument is to set up, 'with the backing of positivist science, a defensive guard which allows us to deny the grip of language on our being' (Flahault, 1978: 36).

This grip is precisely what we have been seeking to make apparent by showing that the subject is formed and exists only in and through speech. Speech is the earth from which we emerge as conscious individuals.

Speech is also a place of 'alienation' in the literal sense of the word, that is, 'a transfer of rights'. Self-realization through speech comes as we receive the *right to speak* from others. And this is a right we can exercise only from the places we are assigned and the places where we are 'recognized'.

In this space, the speaking subject is 'caught' in a web of 'images' having to do with 'who you are for me and who I am for you' (Flahault, 1978: 70), a web that entangles his or her own emerging speech in all sorts of imagined constraints. So here stands the speaker in a place of constant 'birth' where 'he doesn't *become* except as he speaks, that is, as he inevitably takes his place before the image that he believes the other has of him' (Barthes, 1978: 10).

How paradoxical, then, is the situation of the speaker. Placed at the crossroads of two opposing strategies, of liberation and oppression, the speaker goes through a mind-boggling maieutic process to emerge as a 'free subject'.

The subject is both free and constrained even in producing the sounds of speech. The speech sounds we hear ourselves make are not our own except because we have received them, 'drunk them in' like a mother's milk.

So intertwined is verbal activity with the way signifiers sound that their physical qualities sometimes become most important of all. Freud (1960: 119) points out, for instance, that witticisms focus 'our psychical attitude upon the *sound* of the word instead of upon its *meaning*'. As subjects, we free ourselves from signified meanings in order to play with the consonance of the signifiers and to derive real pleasure from them. In doing so, we rediscover an original spontaneity that allows us to freely express ourselves and to explore possible new identities.

If we take the view defended here — that speech is intrinsically linked to the subject — then this playful dimension of language is not a parallel or secondary phenomenon; it is fundamental to the speech process. This playful dimension of language is a place where the speaker, wedged between freedom and dependency, can 'play': it is a place where the question of whose speech is whose does not arise and where the inherent stress of the speaking subject's position disappears.

In light of what has just been summarized, let us take a look at what 'speaking' is for a deaf person.

Although a deaf person's voice may be a little rough and the sounds he or she produces a bit awkward, we readily identify these sounds as words. We do not question the fact that such a person is 'speaking'. But are these words the same as the ones we produce, those of us who are hearing?

Our speech is based on auditory feedback — *speaking is hearing oneself.* Yet profoundly deaf people do not hear at all. Even with a hearing aid their ear cannot pick up the acoustical qualities of speech. This means that they have to rely on a much more complicated kind of feedback, namely the kinesthetic and cenesthetic feel of each articulatory movement painstakingly mastered through years of rigorous childhood training. A deaf person must also figure out how speech sounds are made to flow together to form a sequence of speech. This involves acquiring all of the muscle control and coordination that articulation requires, without being able to rely on 'natural' aural feedback. To do so, the deaf person must be consciously aware of the intricate synergy to be coordinated between breathing, making the vocal cords vibrate, opening and closing the mouth and positioning the tongue and lips.

When we stop to think that each phoneme lasts only some few hundredths of a second, we realize what an incredible feat it is for a deaf person to master speech. In the nineteenth century, educators acknowledged and brought recognition to this astounding achievement by referring to the speech of the deaf as 'artificial'.

In the twentieth century we have tended to ignore this achievement in our eagerness to abolish differences even before truly acknowledging that they exist. Honest acknowledgement of differences unsettles us, unsettles our assumptions and our securities. Yet how can we deal with reality if we don't acknowledge it? How can our actions be effective and appropriate?

We have seen that deaf people produce speech through a process that is physically very different from speech production in hearing people. Now let us consider what a vocal exchange physically requires from the perspective of a deaf person.

On the receiving end, the deaf person perceives the message as a visual image: since sounds cannot reach him, he must refer to the lip and face movements of his interlocutor in order to 'read' his speech. One must realize that this procedure (more accurately called 'speech-reading' than 'lip reading' since the entire face and not just the lips must be 'read') relies heavily on mental guesswork. Only one third of what is said is actually visible on the lips. To be convinced of this, one need only run through the many phonemes that look the same on the lips — [p] [b] [m]; [t] [d] [n]; [f] [v]; etc. — and those that are altogether invisible, such as [k] and [g].

Speech-reading requires great concentration from the deaf person. It is truly possible only when the subject knows the topic of conversation and can reasonably guess at what cannot be grasped through speech-reading alone. In addition, the speaker must be positioned directly in front of the person reading his lips and must speak clearly — not, for example, with a cigarette in his mouth. Mustaches can also get in the way and hide the position of the lips.

Now take a conversation among several people. The deaf person won't be able to follow or participate by speech-reading. First of all, he can't see everyone directly face to face. Secondly, it will take him a few seconds to figure out who is talking each time a different person begins to speak, by which time several words will have already passed him by.

That is what it is like to be on the receiving end of speech when you can't hear. When, in turn, a deaf person is the one sending the message, he must rely on the kinesthetic and vibrating sensations of his own articulatory movements. So, in the course of a spoken interaction, the deaf person receives signs which, for him, are visual, and produces signs recognizable only as kinesthetic sensations. Under such conditions, oral communication becomes a complex process indeed!

How different is a spoken exchange under normal conditions (i. e. when the speakers can hear). Here, the sign never changes in nature. Whether being produced or received, it always remains a message-carrying sound image.

Thus, for a deaf person, spoken interaction is something entirely different from what it is for a hearing person. Nineteenth century educators were sensitive to this fact as well. Joseph-Marie Degérando (1827) addresses this difference in *De l'éducation des sourds-muets de naissance* (educating the congenitally deaf), with the same great sensitivity that he demonstrates throughout the work:

> When a person endowed with hearing speaks or listens, the same sign always serves to interpret thought... But this cannot be said of the lip alphabet and the oral alphabet[4]. Their signs do not belong to the same order of sensations at all; the one arises from sight, the other from touch... This circumstance surely... impairs the effects of empathy. For those of us who are blessed with hearing, the speech of other men is the same as our own. This identity of expression is of singular aid in identifying meaning. We understand each other better. In fact we do more than understand: our minds nearly converge into each other. This intimacy of relation cannot exist for the deaf-mute because the two instruments he uses in alternation are foreign to each other. (Degérando, 1827: 414, 420)

How could one better express what deaf people are denied? Because they cannot perceive sound, even the sound of their own voice, they are effectively excluded from any pleasure in the physical aspects of speech. Sounds are precisely what allow hearing people to communicate, to touch each other, to express and identify themselves; sounds are what offer us a gratuitous space where we can escape the constraints of serious interaction; sounds are what make it possible to play with speech.

One cannot jump from a sound-sign to its double visual-kinesthetic reflection without losing something and upsetting the entire speech process. We must recognize that to speak, deaf people must put out enormous effort and be extremely skilled. Moreover, deaf people can enjoy neither the 'normal' speech process nor the pleasure, play and ease so fundamental to it. Producing and using speech without hearing it may be an admirable skill, but it cannot possibly satisfy a deaf person's needs as a speaking subject.

In other words, speech produced without the natural feedback of sound cannot be the privileged place of self-expression and identification for deaf people that it is for hearing people.

Moreover, using an 'artificial' language can greatly affect a deaf person's ability to '*situate*' him or herself and to *exist* in spoken interactions with hearing people. The following testimony of a 22-year-old woman will help us understand what the deaf person must deal with in such interactions. This young, congenitally deaf woman with a hearing loss of between 80 and 90 dB, learned at a very young age to articulate so correctly that it would take someone a while to realize that she was deaf. Yet here is what she has to say about growing up:

> In play, deafness wasn't a problem. The trouble began when relationships started to revolve around discussions and spoken exchanges. I felt excluded then because no one talked to you 'just for the pleasure of it', but only to transmit a 'practical' message to you... I am uncomfortable in group discussions, even in friendly get-togethers. Even if someone agrees to be the go-between — and I have lots of friends who do — he will only be able to relate the 'skeleton' of the story, which by then has lost all of its flavor. I laugh to please him, but often it's no longer funny or I haven't understood. Everything I get is in the past tense, and I have no way of responding or contributing. (Armengaud, 1979: 266)

We have seen that we really can't speak but from an assigned place and that, as constraining as that place may be, it is nonetheless the place where we are recognized and situated and where we can always enter into greater freedom as speaking subjects. Yet given this woman's story, we must ask ourselves if the deaf person in fact has a place in the spoken interactions in which he or she attempts to participate.

In the absence of hearing, a conversation based on the medium of sound is difficult to follow. Even hearing people experience this difficulty when speaking to a deaf person — how much easier to make oneself understood to another hearing person! This is why hearing people tend to minimize their interaction with the deaf and tend to limit themselves to 'practical' messages rather than converse 'just for the pleasure of it'.

The consequences of this are serious. Because deaf people have difficulty participating in an exchange, they are not recognized as full-fledged partners. As a result, they are excluded from the contact and recognition that form the very basis of linguistic communication between partners to an exchange.

Conclusion: A Way of Seeing Deaf Children

In approaching our subject of speech in deaf children, we have devoted this first chapter to studying the speech process itself. For we cannot determine what our role *vis-à-vis* deaf children should be unless we first answer the question, 'What is speaking?' or 'What are we doing when we speak?'.

The answers to these questions have shown, first, what a complex activity speech really is, and second, that the speech act is something entirely different from the preconceived notions we get from conventional wisdom and sometimes even from university courses colored by the 'platitude of modern information theory' (Lacan, 1977: 305). Our speech can be reduced neither to a simple transparent code nor to an instrument essentially fashioned to transmit information between preexisting subjects.

We cannot disassociate speech from the subject, for the subject comes to exist only in the emergence of his or her own speech. There is no subject but a speaking subject. Speech thus pertains to an entirely different kind of process and thereby loses a good deal of its transparency and innocence.

Speech is not only 'what is said' — a representation — but also an act that the speaking subject takes into account and that reflects back on itself (as shown on page 4). The speech act assumes its full meaning only in terms of the positioning process between the speakers, who are at once formed and limited by the 'who I am for you, and who you are for me' aspect of their speech. But in its sound matter, speech is also a place where the subject can sidestep the stress of serious speech uses and indulge in play (as shown in the section on 'The Speaking Subjects Place in the Speech Process').

These facts force us to recognize how very complex the speech process really is when its phatic, expressive and playful aspects are accepted as fundamental rather than 'deviant', as do over-simplified theories.

For the purposes of our research, recognizing the full complexity of speech means risking a much more complex approach toward deaf children. Yet herein lies the key to progress, for we can apply to teaching what Benveniste (1971, forward) asserts with respect to advances in linguistics: 'Like the other sciences, linguistics advances in direct proportion to the *complexity* which it recognizes in things'.

In presenting two observations of speech production in deaf subjects, we showed that a deaf person can 'speak' — do something which on the outside resembles what we do when we speak — while in reality doing something quite different. In the first case we witnessed a verbal exchange in which a deaf child failed to occupy his 'place' as a speaking subject and thus failed to perform a true speech act. Yet what else can we expect? His teachers had always presented speech as a code. In the second case we saw what enormous physical differences speaking involves depending on whether or not one can hear the sounds of speech. To say that a deaf person 'speaks' means neither that he has complete mastery of the speech process nor that his needs as a speaking subject are satisfied.

Speech is a hard reality with its own laws and requirements. In disregarding or not respecting them because they are not simple, we certainly complicate the lives of the deaf children whom we say we want to teach to speak. We make them pay dearly for our lack of honesty, sometimes jeopardizing their entire equilibrium. The only way that we can better respond to deaf children and free them from our own false assumptions is to adopt an approach that 'recognizes the complexity of things'.

In concluding this chapter, we can now abolish the myth that deaf infants are 'infants without language'. In this view, deaf children are recognized as subjects yet portrayed as 'lacking language'. In defining the speech process, however, we discovered that there can be no such thing as a language-less subject. If deaf children exist as subjects, they necessarily exist as *speaking* subjects.

With respect to language, we tend to think that deaf children are a *tabula rasa*. Yet deaf children can't help but develop language and their own way of speaking. We might not recognize it as such at first, for it will necessarily be quite different from our speech as hearing people. But a *difference in language* is not *an absence of language*. It's simply that we don't have the eyes to recognize the speech that deaf children develop in their ingenuity as speaking subjects. Eager as we are to 'teach' our articulated speech to these little beings, we remain unaware of their own.

Deaf children require that we look at them. How can we see what makes them unique if we don't give them our visual attention, if we don't look at them? Just as an unusual object remains a mystery until carefully observed, so deaf children — unusual in our hearing world — remain misunderstood until we become truly attentive to them. To see deaf children in their own reality we must give them our full attention. When we do, we no longer perceive only what they lack — articulated speech — but come to see them in their own special way of expressing themselves and expressing things to us.

To look at deaf children is to look beyond appearances, to acknowledge their status as full-fledged speaking subjects, and to understand that they cannot achieve verbal communication through the same language modalities that we hearing people use. Our language is meant to be heard and cannot offer the same benefits to a deaf person that it does to a hearing person. But deaf children do try to express themselves in their own way, in a modality that is right for them.

Adopting an approach intended not to evade but to candidly examine the demands of language, thus opens our eyes to how we might accept deaf children in a positive way as speaking subjects. We must not 'make' them speak, but 'let' them speak. We must listen to them and try to respond.

With a view to such acceptance, the following chapter examines how children acquire speech, for deaf children are *infants* just like ordinary children. Whatever ordinary children need to be able to speak, deaf children need as well.

Notes to Chapter 1

1.   The *linguistic sign* is a unit that links a concept (the signified) with its representation (the signifier).
2.   Benveniste uses the term 'statement' in its accepted definition as a unique utterance that is linked to the speaker and the situation in which it is spoken. He disregards the notion of the context-free available sentence.
3.   A violation of a maxim can in fact be explainable if it is done to avoid breaking another rule. For example, if someone answers the question 'What time did John come?' with 'John came in the afternoon', the rule of quantity is violated (not all the expected information is given) in order not to break the rule of quality — if the exact time that John came is not known.
4.   Degérando uses three terms to refer to lipreading and sound production respectively.

2 How Children Acquire Speech

As should be clear from Chapter 1, language is not merely an instrument used to represent and communicate things: it is a complex process in and through which we come to exist as subjects. 'Well before serving to communicate, language serves to live', asserts Benveniste (1974: 217); for, in that it signifies, language establishes the 'possibility of society, the possibility of humanity'. Language is not so much a vehicle for content as a process that brings speakers into relationship.

Babies connect with those around them well before they can talk. They are born into a world of speaking people who talk to them and receive them as future speaking subjects. According to Dominique Weil (1979: 302), the human being is born into a universe where 'language already is, fully formed and supported by speech, which from the outset records each of his relations with others and the elements of his environment'.

Since a child's language history begins at birth, this is where we will begin in observing how children acquire speech in the process of connecting with those around them.

The Newborn's Ability to Communicate

> *We have to feed babies...*
> *We must gorge them with warmth and caresses*
> *just as we do with milk.*
> Frederick Leboyer, *Loving Hands*

Tiny as they may be, babies are social beings right from birth. Just as they are prepared to breathe and nurse, they are also prepared to communicate and connect with others.

Babies are very attentive to human faces and voices. Empirical studies undertaken in the first days of life have revealed that infants, even newborns, react to their mother by crying, seeking skin contact and bodily warmth, following her with their eyes and smiling. Through these innate mechanisms, infants satisfy their need for others. In René Zazzo's (1979) view, smiling can be thought of as

> the motor equivalent of baby birds following behind their mother, or baby monkeys gripping their mother's fur. The human baby, who cannot get around and cannot grip things, is able to establish contact and bonds from a distance by smiling. (Zazzo, 1979: 211)

Human babies are very immature when they enter the world: it takes from eight to ten months for them just to be able to crawl! According to Kenneth Kaye (1977), it is no mistake that our species delivers its young when they are still so immature. This immaturity turns out to be the greatest advantage newborns have: since their behavior is fairly predictable, their mother can learn how to behave with them — provided that she is attentive. A mother is not someone who brings order to chaos, but someone who adapts to the behavior patterns of her baby.

Thus, there seems to be good reason why the most biologically advanced organism is born in such a primitive neurological state: this immaturity fosters between mother[1] and infant the communication and cooperation so essential to all human relationships.

Ashley Montagu's research on babies corroborates these observations. After 266.5 days of gestation, the human foetus, and particularly its head, has grown to such a size that the baby must be born if it is to make it through the birth canal at all. The brain grows so quickly that later, birth would be impossible. But the fact that babies are born after 266.5 days in the womb does not mean that gestation is then complete. Montagu reports that gestation continues outside of the womb. This *exterogestion* is believed to last as long as *uterogestion*; that is, up until the time the child can crawl.

During this second gestation period, infants need intimate contact with their mother. They need

> to be handled, and carried, and caressed, and cuddled, and cooed to... it is the handling, the carrying, the caressing, the caregiving and the cuddling that we would here emphasize, for it would seem that even in the absence of a great deal else, these are the reassuringly basic experiences the infant must enjoy if it is to survive in some semblance of health. (Montagu, 1971: 79)

So great is the newborn's need for contact that 'there is no such thing as an infant', quips Winnicott (1960: 586) in emphasizing that 'the infant and the maternal care together form a unit'. Winnicott takes holding to be an important part of maternal care: 'Holding includes especially the physical holding of the infant, which is a form of loving. It is perhaps the only way in which a mother can show the infant her love of it' (ibid.: 591).

Mother–infant communication first takes place through skin contact and touching. At first this communication occurs in a state of fusion. Because the mother identifies with her newborn, she understands and empathizes with the infant's needs. This is what Winnicott calls 'primary maternal preoccupation'. A mother gets absorbed in her baby — constantly busy nursing it, changing it, carrying it. As the devoted mother tries to adapt to all of her baby's needs, the baby develops a feeling of 'continuity of being' (ibid.: 594).

Winnicott goes on to say that when maternal care goes well it is 'scarcely noticed, and is a continuation of the physiological provision that characterizes the prenatal state' (ibid.: 591). Here we find similarities to Montagu's perspective that gestation does not end at birth. And right along with all this maternal care babies hear their mother's melodic voice: mothers talk to their child right from birth and thus bring him or her into the world as a speaking subject, not as a thing or a baby.

Children hear the voice of their father and mother while still in the womb and must continue to hear these voices after birth. This is a point that Françoise Dolto (1977) insists upon in her approach toward children:

> I believe that the first conversation that a baby has in its mother's arms is very important: 'We've been expecting you, you know. You are a little boy. Perhaps you heard that we were expecting a little girl, but we are very happy that you are a little boy'. (Dolto, 1977: 24)

Dolto emphasizes how important it is to start talking to infants as soon as they are born, for 'all that is put into words becomes human' (ibid.: 25).

Speech brings a certain regularity to children's emotional states: they are constantly spoken to throughout the interactions involved in nursing, eye-contact, etc. When they cry, they are told of their suffering or anger; when they smile, they are told of their well-being and what they like.

As a part of maternal care, speech allows a mother to experience her child not just as an extension of herself, but as an 'other' whom she talks to and receives as a speaking subject. Very early on, this creates moments when 'the mother seems to know that the infant has a new capacity, that of giving a signal so that she can be guided toward meeting the infant's needs' (Winnicott, 1960: 592). These moments become increasingly significant and provide a tiny distance between the expression and satisfaction of need. In other words, they keep children from living in complete symbiosis with their mother. In this tiny distance the notions of time, space and individuality begin to take form for children; they begin to realize that their mother is a separate object from themselves.

In this distance, children's innate behaviors toward others give way to acquired behaviors that are learned in connection with the way their mother responds to them. At first a child's cries are fairly monotone, but by the third or fourth week they begin to modulate, letting the mother recognize a cry of hunger, a cry of strength, a cry of boredom, a cry of wanting to be picked up, or a cry of discomfort. The same is true of smiling, which begins to develop just an hour after birth. It's not long at all before smiling changes in value depending on whether it is intended for the mother or a stranger. In fact, children seem to develop signs of recognition with their mother very quickly — even before they are able to discriminate between her and a stranger or react negatively to her absence.

The first object that exists for children is their primary caretaker — usually their mother. But not long afterward, they become interested in two objects: father and mother. Then, as they grow older, such objects quickly multiply to include additional family members and other familiar people.

Right from birth, children are prepared and equipped to communicate with other human beings. Their behavior commands the attention of those around them: 'Children are treated as subjects who, like anyone, "want" or "don't want" to smile' (Malrieu, 1979: 117). As a mother responds to her child's reaching out, a unique tapestry of interwoven bonds begins to take shape. These patterns, which emerge within the first few months, reflect the mother's own life history from which she has developed 'certain special ways of responding to others, and thus to her child' (ibid.: 117).

But as able communicators, children also transform their parents: we are talking about a deep reaching kind of interaction — a *co-action* between mother and child.

We have already established that speech is an illocutionary act between two or more subjects. Logically, then, we should closely examine the processes of preverbal communication that develop between mother and child right from birth and see if we find in them the beginnings of verbal communication.

Preverbal Communication

Until very recently, language acquisition research consisted essentially in analyzing children's verbal activity at various stages in their development and then trying to write out the grammar underlying their utterances. This is how the linguistic ability of a subject was determined regardless of whether one believed with Chomsky that such ability resulted from an 'innate system of language acquisition' (Language Acquisition Device (LAD)), or with Piaget that it arose out of a whole combination of sensory-motor activities.

Such studies generally traced children's emerging use of the formal aspects of language, rather than how they might use language in various everyday situations. In other words, language was essentially considered only as a code.

But, as we know from Chapter 1, language can hardly be reduced to a code. By neglecting the practical dimension of speech, researchers missed their mark: they never explained how language is acquired. Consequently, their studies also contributed little to our understanding of what readies a child for speech acquisition.

Today's trend in research focuses more closely on the communicative function and semantic aspects of language. In his study on the prelinguistic prerequisites of speech, Jerome Bruner (1978) poses the question of language within the larger framework of communication processes in general, from which language results. Whereas language may be the primary and most significant result of the communication process, it is still just that — a result.

Calling upon the work of ordinary-language philosophers, Bruner argues that speech prerequisites are to be found *in children's preverbal interaction with their mother*. In Bruner's view, the crucial component of any language acquisition process lies in the connection between the illocutionary act of an utterance and its syntactic form. This connection between 'the fact of speaking', 'the act of speaking', and 'what is said' — to use the terms we presented earlier — is what apparently enables children to pick up language so quickly.

As a mother and child become jointly engaged in their first social interactions, a whole combination of little rituals begins to develop by mutual agreement. Through this play, this expression of culture, children discover the mechanisms of *dialogue*, *reference* and *predication*, and thus acquire an understanding of the underlying rules of linguistic activity. Let us examine these three mechanisms in language.

The emergence of dialogue in joint mother–infant activity

From the moment her baby opens its eyes and looks at her, a mother can't possibly react as she would toward an inanimate object. She immediately seeks to interact with her baby through ritualized social exchanges, and very quickly the infant begins to take part. *Social* beings right from birth, infants are also *cultural* beings.

Innovative film and video techniques have made it possible to observe early mother–infant interactions in greater detail than ever before. Slow-motion, synchronized playback has revealed new phenomena and made clear the distinctions between what comes from the mother and what comes from the infant during an exchange. These newly observable facts are highly significant to our hypothesis of continuity between preverbal and verbal communication.

We have seen that the devoted mother adapts to her infant's behavior. She responds to the baby's smiles, looks, cries and need for contact. A mother in fact responds to her baby's gestures and actions as though they were intended to communicate something. This is not yet dialogue, but *pseudo-dialogue*, for it is always up to the mother to furnish a 'response'. But a mother's very anticipation of her baby's communication potential serves to restructure and develop the infant's behavior along two parallel processes: reciprocity and intentionality — both of which are well established by the twelfth month, that is, before verbal communication begins.

In his systematic study of mother–infant interaction, John Newson (1977) pays careful attention to the way in which mothers set up interaction sequences 'as if' the process were reciprocal by acting in perfect sync with whatever their child is doing. Mothers catch on to the rhythm of their infant's activity and use natural pauses to insert their own reaction — usually managing to avoid any overlap at all.

Mothers display a great deal of sensitivity in listening to their baby so that they can fine-tune their own behavior to his or hers. Hanuš and Mechthild Papoušek (1977) have shown that in addition to being attentive to their infant's expressions, smiles, sounds and body language, mothers also clue into very subtle signals, such as hand and finger positions that indicate whether their infant is awake and attentive, uncomfortable or sleepy.

Only when a mother senses her infant's attention will she initiate an interaction — always based on the child's own spontaneous actions. This behavior allows infants to become increasingly aware of their mother's interest in their activity and realize that she is attentive and will respond to what they do. Infants are able to make this discovery all the more easily given that maternal responses are arranged in repetitive and ritualized routine sequences that let them more or less predict their mother's behavior. Infants delight in such interactions: their mother's response provides the desired result and gives them the satisfaction of being able to control events insofar as they can predict them. Eventually, this ability to predict a particular behavior entices infants to initiate the exchange themselves. Having realized that their mother paid attention to their behavior and that it produced certain results, infants will initiate the dialogue in order to elicit the expected response. At this point they become a complete partner to a true dialogue, a dialogue that will let them discover the rules behind taking turns. Thus emerges the basic procedure for all linguistic communication.

The few empirical observations that follow illustrate how dialogue gradually develops between mother and infant.

In a research project involving 30 newborns between 2 and 18 days old, Kenneth Kaye (1977) studied burst–pause patterns during nursing and observed how mothers and infants each react. He found that mothers behave differently depending on whether their baby is sucking or has stopped. When babies pause, mothers tend to jiggle them more and take the nipple (be it a bottle's or the mother's own) out of their mouth to gently tap it on their lips. While babies are sucking, however, these behaviors are much less frequent.

Contrary to what mothers believe, jiggling does not make a baby begin sucking again any sooner; in fact it seems to delay resumption. Kaye observed a change in this mother–infant interaction over time from the second day to the second week: mothers tend to reduce the duration of their jiggling during pauses. It is as if they subconsciously realize that jiggling doesn't help. Instead of 'jiggling until sucking begins', they 'jiggle and stop'. So something of a rule develops that is simultaneously learned by the mother and her newborn: 'Now it's your turn, now its my turn'. According to Kaye, this is the first observable example of turn-taking being learned in the mother–infant relationship.

In a study on imitation interactions, Susan Pawlby (1977) showed how mother and infant learn to switch roles and establish dialogue. The fact that mothers tend to imitate certain gestures or sounds that their baby makes and attribute communicative value to these activities right from birth is nothing new. But Pawlby made the rather striking discovery that when mothers see that their infant is going to repeat one particular spontaneous action two or three times in a kind of repetitive ritual, they cleverly insert their own repetitions between their baby's in syncopation. Mothers thereby create a sequence of repetitions in which the infant appears to imitate *them*. This kind of pseudo-imitation and *pseudo-dialogue* lets mothers maintain their illusions about their infant's communication abilities and show their desire to continue these meaningful interactions. Mothers thus tend to ritualize their own imitation behavior toward their baby.

The particular gestures, faces and sounds that a mother regularly imitates will become important and hold special meaning for her baby. By imitating her baby in this way, a mother offers him or her a sort of 'biological mirror' (Papoušek and Papoušek, 1977: 82). Babies show how much these imitations delight them by laughing or smiling. What the infant first produced spontaneously, he or she will attempt to repeat more deliberately, specifically to elicit the mother's imitation. This kind of dialogue sequence initiated by the infant can be observed as early as the sixth month. Sometimes they involve not just one, but several different exchanges that follow one after the other until one partner loses the other's attention.

A mother's knowing just how to repeat her imitations and how to adjust them to her baby's rhythms greatly aid the infant in discovering his or her own power of prediction and eventually draw the child into *true* dialogue.

Pawlby's research, based on observations of eight different mothers playing freely with their respective babies during the 17 to 43-week-old period, showed that mothers are not really aware of their behavior or of the fact that they are providing their baby with a framework so sophisticated and advantageous that it brings about true dialogue. They are aware only of the fact that their baby imitates *them*. Little do they realize that this imitation behavior follows initial exchanges in which they were the ones who imitated their baby. 'Paradoxically', writes Pawlby (1977: 219), 'our study suggests that the whole process by which the infant comes to imitate his mother in a clearly intentional way is rooted in the initial readiness of the *mother* to imitate her infant'.

Bruner (1977: 283) has conducted similar research on give-and-take situations. In a longitudinal study including data on 20 mothers with their 3 to 15 month-old infants he shows how behaviors of reciprocity and intentionality develop in infants. When giving games begin at around three months, they can hardly be considered an 'exchange': it is up to the mother to make it all happen. A mother knows that a brightly colored, noisy object such as a rattle, will most easily catch her infant's interest and attention. She will jiggle it right in front of her baby at an appropriate distance and simultaneously encourage him or her with faces and verbal coaxing. By her exaggerated and drawn out manner she will eventually get her baby to take the object. In her mind, it is as though the infant has taken it deliberately.

In trying to give something to her baby, a mother will first limit her offerings to a single object. Sometimes she will press it into her baby's hand herself, only to have the infant let it drop. There ends the exchange. But the mother will continue to try, starting all over again.

When the baby is about six months old, this mother–infant activity begins to resemble a real exchange in which the infant 'takes' the object in a more intentional way. At this point, the mother doesn't have to be so animated to catch her infant's attention, and she can succeed in offering him or her a variety of different objects. Now the infant directs his or her attention more squarely on the object and will 'take' it, without relying so much on the mother's prompting.

If her infant lets it fall, as often happens, the mother waits for him or her to pick it up if it is within reach.

At this stage, the give-and-take interaction is still very rudimentary. The infant may 'take' things, but only in a very simplistic manner: the infant doesn't yet reciprocate the action by then 'giving'. Yet through this kind of interaction the infant eventually discovers the reciprocity of the game. By the time the infant is around 12 months old he or she is able to fully participate, trading off being the giver and the taker.

These three examples of mother–infant activity — nursing, imitation and give-and-take — make it clear that infants are involved in highly ritualized interaction with their mother right from birth. Because it is so regular and well-adapted, a mother's behavior provides a framework that will help her baby master the rules of turn-taking and thereby enter into true dialogue. How could language even develop in a child who hasn't learned these rules so basic to it?

The above examples also reveal the atmosphere of play and pleasure in which conventions and rules are established and dialogue develops. Such an atmosphere appears to be another very important condition for language development. Bruner considers such harmony and pleasure to be a *sine qua non* necessity: 'when things become too "serious", and intention-bound, communication regresses to the level of demand and counter demand' and loses its flavor as a game — and games are what create bonds and understandings on multiple levels (Bruner, 1977: 288).

This climate of play and pleasure will continue to be an important focus throughout our study as we trace the transition from play to personal identity, '*du jeu au je*' as Jean-Baptiste Pontalis puts it in his preface to the French edition of Winnicott's *Playing and Reality* (1975).

The following section examines how preverbal communication leads the infant to discover reference and how it works.

Discovering reference and how it works through joint mother–infant attention

Very young infants are interested mainly in human beings, but after a few months the inanimate world also begins to capture their interest and visual attention. As it does, material objects in their environment begin to play an important part in mother–infant interactions.

Research carried out by Glyn Collis and H. R. Schaffer (1975) shows that in certain circumstances, and beginning at birth, mothers continually follow their infant's eye-gaze, even if what the infant is looking at has nothing to do with their interaction. Experiments conducted by Scaife and Bruner (1975) further reveal that as early as age four months, infants sometimes follow the eye gaze of an adult when the adult turns to look at something in the distance. This ability increases rapidly and demonstrates a measure of decentring in that the infant can follow another person's gaze and share in his or her interest. Mothers often notice this development at about six months, unaware that they have been following their infant's eye-gaze all along and were initially the one responsible for their mother–infant visual co-orientation.

Infants learn that they can show what interests them in other ways as well: holding out and showing an object, hitting it against something, making certain sounds, etc.

Bruner (1977: 275) sees in this behavior the beginnings of referential activity. He suggests that, for infants, reference is not a matter of linking a particular gesture, face or sound with an object, but of singling out a particular object from the whole array of things around them.

Referential activity begins with being able to indicate clearly to another person which object or action out of many is the specific focus of the exchange. Bruner calls this the 'efficacy of singling out'. Infants display great creative abilities in this discovery process, which they apply not to just one kind of object but to absolutely everything in their little world.

The way in which infants single out objects of interest changes rapidly. At first they resort to a whole combination of postures, gestures and vocalizations, impatiently trying to reach for the object. Gradually they adopt more efficient means that are less dependent on context. By about eight months, infants sharing an attentive moment with their mother will merely hold out a hand toward an object to express their interest in it instead of displaying impatience as before. Meanwhile, they search their mother's face to see if she understands the meaning of their gesture. This new approach more closely resembles conventional reference techniques.

As a longitudinal study by Ninio and Bruner (1978) shows, infants use these newly acquired signaling techniques first as a means of reference and eventually as a basis for labeling. Specifically, Ninio and Bruner regularly observed a mother–infant dyad engaged in free play from age 8 to 18 months. During exchanges centered around a picture-book, the infant would smile, reach, point or make babbling vocalizations in an attempt to point out images as they became the object of joint mother–infant attention. The mother would interpret these behaviors as attempts by her infant to label what he saw. Not insignificantly, these first 'labeling' behaviors first occurred in connection with a picture-book: pictures are nothing other than two-dimensional representations of three-dimensional objects. Infants seem to resolve this conflict quite quickly by understanding pictures as objects that can't be held. In fact, it is when sitting with a picture-book that infants most often resort to pointing rather than grabbing to designate something. 'This process might be one of the stepping stones to grasping arbitrary symbolic representation in language, since visual representations are themselves arbitrary in the sense that a crucial object property, i. e. graspability, is missing' (Ninio and Bruner, 1978: 5).

The picture-book was used as the starting point for ritualized mother–infant dialogues similar to this one, recorded when the child was 13 months old (ibid.: 6):

Mother: Look! (ATTENTIONAL VOCATIVE)
Child: (Touches picture)
M: What are those? (QUERY)
C: (Vocalizes and smiles)
M: Yes, they are rabbits. (FEEDBACK[2] AND LABEL)
C: (Vocalizes, smiles and looks up at mother)
M: (Laughs) Yes, rabbit. (FEEDBACK AND LABEL)
C: (Vocalizes, smiles)
M: Yes (laughs) (FEEDBACK)
(ibid.: 6)

It was the mother who would elicit the labeling by offering a very structured and highly repetitive framework. She always began every 'reading' period in the same way: 'Look!' or 'What's that?'. Also, the mother always offered feedback on the child's vocalizations before giving the name of the thing the picture represented. Before offering a model to imitate, the mother encouraged the child's own spontaneous expression. In doing so, she anticipated the child's ability to label things himself.

The above sample dialogue illustrates how much both partners enjoyed this interaction. Once children are able to approximate the 'correct' form of various words, they begin to name things and people just for the pleasure of it — including the pleasure of being able to draw someone's attention to a particular object out of the entire surroundings. In other words, children don't begin labeling for any practical purpose such as obtaining something or communicating a message. They engage in labeling in order to prolong the very pleasurable experience of joint attention. Labeling also lets children show that they can link a 'name' with its referent. By naming things, children discover a new relationship with the world. According to Heinz Werner and Bernard Kaplan (1963), the world becomes a set of objects to be contemplated, not just manipulated. This development becomes a factor in the overall 'separation' process by which children establish themselves as subjects *vis-à-vis* their mother and the world.

Once we closely examine how mothers usher their children into this naming process, and once we discover how clever and apt their strategy is, we can't help but realize that it is rather ridiculous to think, as many do, that language naturally develops by itself. Mothers may not be fully aware of the techniques that they are using, and these techniques may be a source of shared joys and well-being, but nonetheless the child is being *taught*. This is a fact that we must not ignore, regardless of how 'hardly noticeable' it may be — just like a mother's care when all goes well.

In short, and as Bruner has substantiated, the idea of giving things names quite clearly dawns on children well before they are able to talk.

Now let us turn to predication techniques and observe how children discover them through playful exchanges with their mother.

Discovering predication techniques through mother–infant interaction

Predication consists in establishing a link between a topic and a comment. The topic is the person or thing about which something is said. The comment is what is said about that particular person or thing.

Among other authors, David McNeill (1970) maintains that a child's holophrastic vocalizations can be seen as comments on an extra-linguistic topic. Bruner goes further to say that joint mother infant activity provides an implicit topic about which comments are made. He suggests that the first and most simple form of commentary involves confirming that a joint activity (the topic) is being shared. Babies do this by interrupting the flow of interaction to smile and look deeply into their mother's eyes before resuming the activity at hand. In this case, the topic is the joint activity and the comment is this confirmation that the topic is in fact being shared by both mother and infant. The infant's look makes the comment: we are both '"with it", engaged in the game' (Bruner, 1977: 280).

Bruner has observed that along with this kind of comment, nine-month-old babies make vocalizations, which he describes as 'proclamative'. They occur only at specific moments during the interaction: when the infant is ready to take his or her turn or upon completing the task. They seem to proclaim such comments as 'it's my turn' or 'it's done'. This type of comment vocalization is particularly noticeable during interactions when both mother and child are doing something with a particular object. Vocalizations either precede or coincide with the infant's look toward his or her mother. Babies also sometimes enhance their vocalizations and visual contact by holding out the object for their mother to see.

For there to be predication, that is, a topic–comment correlation, the topic and comment must be separable. A child's interaction with the physical world leads to this topic–comment separability, suggests Bruner. A child can play with a single object in many different ways: mouth on it, squeeze it, bang it, throw it, grab it. In this case, the object becomes the topic, and what the infant does with it, the comment. Children can also carry out the same action with many different objects. For instance, they can bang a spoon, a cup, a rattle, a doll, etc. Here the single action can be taken as the topic, and the different objects as comments.

Thus in the second six months of life, children are well on their way to discovering the concepts of 'things' and 'properties' in an extra-linguistic sense. They need to understand these notions in order to acquire the predication techniques involved in joint mother–infant activities.

As a final note, we must keep in mind how important eye *contact* is to making comments on an implicit theme.

Summary and pedagogical implications: from play to the speaking subject

If we consider speech within the context of interpersonal relationships rather than as a behavior by a single individual, we have no choice but to acknowledge the wealth of communication that passes between mother and infant *preverbally*.

Only recently have researchers begun to explore and examine preverbal communication and discover the importance of ritualized mother–infant exchanges. These interaction are what draw infants into dialogue.

Well before they can speak, children engage in interactions that require all of the basic characteristics of verbal dialogue: turn-taking, reference techniques and an understanding of predication. This is probably why children seem to develop verbal communication so smoothly and quickly when all goes well — we begin preparing them for it as soon as they are born!

Babies are born with instincts that help them satisfy their need for others. By adapting and adjusting their own behavior to their baby's, mothers are able to weave these instincts into a tapestry of interactions that will develop and modify them. Preverbal communication involves multiple channels that can function simultaneously in a personally unique synchrony. Schaffer, Collis and Parsons (1977) have shown, for example, that infants can coordinate looking at their mother and making vocalizations.

This is a multi-sensory kind of communication that involves looking, smiling, crying, vocalizing, touching, making faces and gesturing. We could even say that anything babies do and any of their senses can become a means of communicating with their mother. This potential vastly increases the range of messages infants can transmit or receive.

Without fully realizing it, mothers supply their infant with a structured and ritualized framework that allows their child's communicative abilities to develop. Anticipating these abilities, mothers accept anything their baby does as though it were intended to communicate something. In the joy of their 'anticipatory illusion' — to use Diatkine's expression (1975: 13) — mothers create the conditions for true dialogue. Before long (at around six months) dialogue fully emerges as the infant becomes capable of initiating ritualized interactions him or herself.

We would thus join those authors who speak of a mother's 'implicit pedagogy'. Here is its golden rule: *in the pleasure of anticipating children's communicative abilities, welcome everything they offer and try to respond in the most appropriate way possible.*

Mothers always structure their own actions around those of their infant. In so doing, they set up *real teaching situations* so gradual and appropriate that they enable the child to cross the threshold of reciprocity and intentionality in communication. What precision and art this requires! And the more these leaps in communication become a source of shared joy and pleasure, the more mother and infant revel in success.

So what would be work becomes *play* — something inconceivable without the pleasure it brings. Yet this implicit maternal pedagogy, this pedagogy of play, is no less a genuine pedagogy as defined by Jean Foucambert (1976: 21): 'Serious pedagogy begins when the schoolmaster shapes his activities to those of the child, when teaching begins with learning'. This is the very approach that mothers discover spontaneously when all goes well, that is, provided that they are psychologically in a state that allows them to be attentive to their infant.

Language does indeed begin at birth. Through playful, pleasurable interactions, mothers bring their infant to respond to them, to 'talk' to them, to become a speaking subject and an active partner in dialogue well before the child ever utters his or her first word.

The great differences in verbal communication skills that exist among ordinary children undoubtedly originate in this opening chapter of each child's language history. These differences — apparent even in three to four-year-old preschoolers — have been a focus of attention for Diatkine as a child psychoanalyst. A child whose first attempts to communicate have not been welcomed or integrated into a meaningful system will not develop to his or her potential. Nor will the child discover the features of preverbal communication that lead to the mastery of all sorts of 'perceptive, motor, conceptual, social *and* linguistic skills' (Bruner, 1975: 256). Incidentally, this is why we speak of *preverbal* rather than *prelinguistic* communication: linguistic skills begin to develop in children before they begin to talk.

If children's first communication attempts are not gratified, their potential for communication will not just go undeveloped — they may lose it altogether. Having seen as much, Diatkine challenges the very popular idea and educational maxim that all school-age children want to communicate. This may be a reassuring assertion, but it does not reflect reality. Diatkine cautions,

> We must not assume... that the need to communicate is universal and natural in all children. I would even say that I am convinced of the contrary... *Petits bourgeois* that we are, we may find it unthinkable that many children don't desire to read, to write or even to talk. But such is reality. (Diatkine, 1973: 136)

These are children in whom the aptitude for communication has been snuffed out. As social beings right from birth, children are also cultural beings who cannot blossom unless others respond to them and interact with them in a highly ritualized manner.

How crucial then is early preverbal communication!

Enormous differences in speech acquisition have also been observed among deaf children: contrary to what one might expect, hearing loss does not dictate a child's level of achievement. It is entirely possible for a profoundly deaf child to be able to communicate more effectively through speech than a child with less hearing loss, even if the two are equally acute intellectually and have benefited from similar speech training. Of course, many different factors can account for these differences, but we are convinced that what passes between a deaf infant and his or her mother during the preverbal stage of communication plays a major role in the child's future speaking ability. What we recognize as essential for hearing children is even more crucial for deaf children. This is a point we will further explore in the conclusion to this chapter.

When professional educators run into communication and language problems, they would do well to take as their model the implicit pedagogy that mothers demonstrate in preverbal communication with their infant. Unfortunately, this process is often examined only superficially, and hence misunderstood as contradictory. The teaching situations mothers provide are so well adapted to their infant's abilities that they create an atmosphere of shared fun and pleasure.

In conventional pedagogy — a pedagogy insufficiently defined by what children put forth — teaching and pleasure are not notions that belong together. Various theories of language development emphasizing either one or the other reflect this dichotomy.

On the one hand, theories that emphasize pleasure declare that 'language is learned but not taught'.[3] In other words, children have to do all the work while adults just talk, talk, talk. This philosophy has even been advocated as a 'new method'[4] for teaching language to deaf children. We can well imagine its damaging effects — it totally disregards the fact that adults must adapt their behavior to that of the child.

On the other hand, theories that emphasize teaching don't take the child's abilities as their starting point either. Children are 'taught' as though they were a *tabula rasa*: no consideration is given to how children actually learn and acquire what we would want to teach them.

Both educational approaches miss their mark. The first proposes pleasure yet offers none, for pleasure comes from children's deep satisfaction at being able to do what they are invited to try. The second advocates teaching yet does not really teach since it neglects what children put forth. So neither approach duplicates the marvelous synthesis that mothers create in communicating with their infant. Through play — teaching that brings pleasure — mothers bring their child into his or her own as a speaking subject.

In preverbal communication children 'speak' before they talk. So what prompts their first words? Why do children suddenly 'speak up'? These are the questions we will be answering as we now examine verbal communication.

Verbal Communication

As we all know, the burgeoning of verbal communication is not as predictable as other more maturity-related developments such as gripping and walking. Sometimes it seems that those first words will never come in certain children even though they already have down the basics of verbal communication, that is, they have the skills to:

(1)   make predictions by distinguishing means from ends,
(2)   accomplish ritualized tasks by following rules,
(3)   communicate intentionally in reciprocity, and
(4)   get others to do what they want them to by ensuring uptake of their messages — i. e. their intentions are well received or understood by others.

According to Bruner (1978: 201), these four skills constitute 'the foundation upon which the child's language acquisition will be constructed'. Yet some children who have sufficiently mastered them still don't seem to want to talk. They don't begin communicating through speech even though verbal communication would accomplish the same functions that they developed in preverbal communication. Then one day, a day no one can predict, such children utter those long-awaited first words. What happened? Why did this new form of communication emerge? What triggered it?

As Bruner admits, the answers to these questions are not entirely clear. We will attempt to explain this transition from preverbal to verbal communication by drawing upon psychoanalytic theory on how children develop psychically. But first we must take account of the fact that children understand what is said to and around them well before they ever speak themselves — particularly when this talk has to do with them. Language comprehension precedes language use. Let us take a look at how this comprehension first develops through mother–infant interaction.

How mothers talk to their child

Mothers talk to their infant right from birth and accompany most of their interactions with words. Mothers don't wait to speak to their baby until he or she can speak back and certainly not until their baby truly communicates intentionally. Right from the start, mothers interpret their baby's reactions as expressions of need or desire: my baby cries 'to say' that he is wet or hungry; my infant looks at an object because she 'wants' it. This attitude leads mothers to converse regularly with their child well before he or she can talk.

Just as we did with respect to preverbal communication, we will now take a close look at how mothers behave when they communicate with their infant verbally. These observations will help us to better understand how children begin to speak.

Establishing Conversation

We have seen that mothers quickly set up preverbal dialogue situations in which their infant can participate and share — even at six months old. We find that mothers exhibit similar behavior when talking to their infant. As Catherine Snow (1978) has shown, they immediately establish a conversational process. To use her example:

A mother who holds up a mobile and says to her child 'Isn't that pretty?' may be equally convinced that communication has occurred by a response of looking at the mobile from a 3-month-old, reaching for it by a 6-month-old, or saying 'Pretty' by an 18-month-old. (Snow, 1978: 256)

By asking questions, mothers create a context in which a whole series of behaviors in their infant can be interpreted as a response. Mothers thus bring about an exchange that gives them the illusion that their child is responding to them and being an effective partner in conversation — even verbally.

This attitude is very important: 'It is to a large extent the experience of having successfully communicated with a child which convinces one that effective communication is possible' (Snow, 1978: 268). This experience is also what encourages mothers to persevere in conversing verbally with their infant.

A mother's anticipatory illusions about the possibility of communicating with her child obviously must be fed by the baby's reactions. Mothers thus try to create situations that will evoke a response. They don't wait until their child can converse to make conversation. They ask questions and then interpret the 'response', be it a look, a nod, a sound or any other reaction by the child to the situation in which the question was posed. As in the above example of a mother asking a question while holding up a mobile, these situations always involve a complex combination of stimuli. Often mothers will even verbalize their own interpretation of the child's 'responses', in this way creating questions and answers.

To do all of this, however, mothers must receive some sort of message from their child. Selma Fraiberg (1974) notes that mothers sometimes find it difficult to converse with a blind baby. They don't know how to interpret the baby's signs of attention or interest because these behaviors don't match those that they expect as sighted individuals. If a mother can't sense or recognize her baby's 'responses', she may become unable to converse with her infant at all.

So even though conversation is carried on entirely by the mother, it is nonetheless based on the child's reactions. Here again we find interaction, or co-action.

Obviously, the mother must enjoy and be interested in talking with her baby if such conversation is to be established. Unfortunately, this is not always the case. A mother's own mental disposition as well as certain social and cultural conditions can dampen her interest. If a mother is exhausted by closely spaced pregnancies or is overextended at work, she may not be able or want to indulge in such apparently gratuitous conversational exchanges. A mother under psychological duress can also lose the feeling and desire for conversing with her baby.

Such may be the case when a mother is informed that her child is deaf. Before deafness is diagnosed, the mother carries on satisfying conversations with her deaf baby that produce the kind of responses she expects — eye gaze, appropriate motor movements, smiles, etc. So important is eye contact to these first exchanges that the mother may not even suspect that her child is deaf. She thus goes along feeding her anticipatory illusions which are so essential to mother–infant conversation. But the discovery of deafness often punctures this illusion — 'Why talk to him if he can't hear me?' — and consequently deprives the child of the atmosphere of communication in which everything he or she did was accepted as a 'statement'.

We will come back to this critical turn of events in the conclusion to this chapter, but let us first examine the mother's speech itself. We have seen that under normal conditions mothers 'converse' with their baby right from birth, creating all of the conditions necessary to a conversation. What makes maternal speech unique?

The special child-directed speech register

When a mother talks to her baby she speaks in a register that is phonologically, syntactically, semantically and discursively different from her normal speech register.

A mother doesn't talk to her infant in the same way she would to other adults or to an older child who can talk. Having observed twenty different languages and dialects, Charles Ferguson (1977: 209) concluded that 'in all speech communities, there are probably special ways of talking to young children which differ more or less systematically from the more "normal" form of the language used in ordinary conversations among adults'.

One universal property of language is that it varies according to use. The speech register used by mothers when addressing their young child constitutes one of these variations. Yet not until the 1960s did researchers really begin to focus on this maternal register. Since then researchers have clearly identified what specifically characterizes this register, particularly as observed in mother–infant exchanges.

Phonological features. The prosody of a mother's speech is different when she speaks to her child from when she speaks with adults. By 'prosody' we mean all of the 'musical elements of language' (Bally, 1932: 79) created by stress, rhythm and intonation. These elements correspond to various physical speech parameters — intensity, duration and voice tone frequency. Each of these features undergoes significant change when a mother talks to her baby. Olga

Garnica (1977) has isolated six different prosodic traits that appear to be specific properties of maternal speech:

(1)   higher fundamental pitch
(2)   frequent rising final pitch terminals, even at the end of non-interrogative utterances
(3)   expanded frequency range from 'normal' speech; sometimes bordering on the sing-songy
(4)   use of whispering
(5)   increased primary stress
(6)   slower speech rhythm.
       (Garnica, 1977)

Garnica's observations indicate that mothers generally exaggerate the prosodic features of their speech and that they apparently do so in order to draw their child's attention and give the infant a cue that he or she is being addressed. The prosodic characteristics of a mother's speech do make it easy to distinguish from the background sounds of adult conversation. The mother's prosody might also serve to make her speech clearer: it divides sequences into more perceptible units. Increased intonation and stress make it easier to recognize the beginning and end of sentences, and word groups within them.

Mothers use these prosodic devices more or less consciously in their effort to guarantee communication with their child at any cost. Understandably, these features evolve as the child grows older. Prosodic exaggeration is most pronounced in the preverbal period when a child's attention span is limited but all of his or her senses are wide awake. By the age of five years, however, this exaggeration decreases significantly.

It is a well recognized fact that most children reproduce intonation patterns long before they speak their first words. They are able to understand and produce distinct intonation patterns that indicate a command, relief, joy or discontent. This explains why children often sound as if they are speaking even though no single word can be identified in their babbling.

Children are also very sensitive to the rhythm of speech. Adults of every culture recognize and respond to this sensitivity with songs, nursery rhymes, lullabies, and children's poems.

There are other phonological features of maternal speech that relate not to prosody but to lexical units. In choosing which words she will use in speaking with her child, a mother tends to use disyllables that follow a consonant–vowel–consonant–vowel pattern. Of all possible lexemes, these are the easiest to articulate and recognize.

Whether prosodic or lexical, all of these phonological features are suited to the sensory and motor capabilities of young children and are found in all languages.

Semantic features. The most prominent semantic feature of maternal speech seems to be that it is always rooted in the here-and-now of the exchange situation. A mother talks about things that are interesting and familiar to her baby. Her speech is therefore very dependent upon context, as will be the child's. At first, a child's speech can be understood only in its immediate context against the backdrop of common mother–infant knowledge.

Snow and Ferguson (1977) discuss this semantic feature as follows:

> Mothers make very predictable comments about very predictable topics, which is precisely what must happen if Macnamara (1972) is correct in his suggestion that children are able to learn to talk because they can work out the meaning of the sentences they hear independent of the sentences themselves. (Snow and Ferguson, 1977: 41)

Snow cites this observation as one reason why she favors language acquisition theories that emphasize the semantic aspects of language.

Among other authors, Marilyn Shatz and Rochel Gelman (1977) point out that changes in child-directed speech are largely a function of what can be talked about given the child's cognitive development. Content modification is at least as significant as changes in how things are said. In fact our manner of speaking may change depending on what we are talking about. Speech is most heavily shaped by our concern with being understood. This is why mothers use simple vocabulary, keeping their messages brief, intelligible and well-formed.

Syntactic features. Utterances aimed at young children are often much shorter than usual. Elissa Newport *et al.* (1977) calculated the average length of mothers' statements to their 12 to 27-month-old children at 4. 24 words, as compared to 11. 94 words when speaking to the experimenter. Mothers know that if they talk for too long they will lose their child's attention. This seems to be why they abbreviate their utterances so severely.

Newport *et al.* also point out that mothers speak with a high level of intelligibility. Only 4% of what they said to their child during this study could not be heard and transcribed for reasons of excessive drops or booms in the voice. This rate reached 9% in conversations with the adult. Mothers make their vocal utterances clearer by slowing their pace and accentuating word-group and sentence boundaries. Moreover, their utterances are always well formed: only one out of 1,500 utterances contained an error in word order. This is infinitesimal compared to the error rate found in conversations among adults, even given the fact that our daily language isn't as full of poor sentences as we might think. In the course of his research, William Labov (1970) discovered that only 2% of the utterances he sampled were non-grammatical. Since the incidence of error in maternal speech is so much lower still, are we to assume that mothers use extremely simplified syntax to converse with their child?

According to Newport *et al.* it would be wrong to say that maternal utterances show 'syntactic simplicity'. As a matter of fact, only 30% of their utterances are declarative as compared to 87% among adults. Furthermore, 72% of maternal utterances involve some sort of optional movement or deletion transformation, as against just 45% in 'normal' speech.

Given these findings, we cannot equate brevity with syntactic simplicity. Even though mothers usually speak in discrete propositions without embedding them in each other or connecting them with conjunctions, this doesn't mean that the individual propositions don't contain syntactic complexities. Interrogatives and imperatives are rarely used in inter-adult speech but frequently appear in maternal speech at a rate of 44% and 18% respectively.

It thus appears that out of a desire to be understood, mothers are more concerned with simplifying the transmission of their message (adapting it to the cognitive abilities of their small child by making it brief, intelligible and well-formed) than with how they structure their syntax. Mothers in fact use a greater variety of syntactic constructions than usual when talking with their children. They practice 'processing simplicity not syntactic simplicity' (Newport *et al.*, 1977: 127).

All of the above goes to show that, above all, mothers seek to *communicate* with their child by taking his or her abilities into consideration rather than attempt to teach their child syntax through graded lessons.

Discursive features. David J. Messer (1980) analyzed maternal speech patterns in a research project involving 42 mothers with their 11 to 24-month-old children. He found that maternal speech is very redundant for the situations in which it occurs. Mothers divide their speech into what Messer calls *verbal episodes*, that is, strings of successive utterances which all refer to the same object. For example:

Episode B:

(3)	oh there's a super car		M brings car to C
(4)	you like cars don't you?		both hold it
(5)	what are you going to do with it?		
(6)	are you going to make it go?		child retains
	(Messer, 1980: 33)		

Mothers repeatedly refer to the object at hand by using names (utterances 3 and 4) or pronouns (utterances 5 and 6). In all such episodes we also find that mothers use the same kinds of sentences over and over again, limiting themselves to questions, statements and imperatives.

The boundaries between verbal episodes are marked by a longer pause than between utterances belonging to the same episode. A new episode rarely begins until the toy to be discussed has been handled. Also, at least the first utterance of an episode generally contains the name of the object that will be referred to throughout. Here, for example, is the episode that followed the previous one:

Episode C:

(7) that's a bus   child picks bus up
(8) bus   both hold
(9) you've got one
      (ibid.: 33)

The older the child gets — the children in this study go up to two years old — the less marked the boundaries between verbal episodes tend to become. The new object is not always manipulated beforehand, nor is it necessarily named at the beginning of the verbal episode.

In observing how mothers carry on discussions with their child and how these discussions evolve, we once again find that same striking quality that characterizes maternal behavior in general: sensitivity to the child's reactions. Maternal verbal behavior is also highly ritualized, just as it is in preverbal communication. In this way, mothers let their child experiment with making predictions — even about speech itself.

Many authors have brought up *repetition*[5] as a significant feature of maternal speech. Jean Berko Gleason (1977) believes repetition is connected with feedback: a mother repeats herself until she receives the expected feedback from her child, be it a slight nod, a look, a gesture or some other signal. Gleason also notes that mothers continue to repeat themselves even after they have received perfectly clear feedback from the child. The following examples illustrate this phenomenon:

Child: (Points to book with crayon) Uh.
Mother: (Nods) Book. Book.
Child: (Grabs book)
Mother: See the book?

Mother: Get the ball.
Child: (Picks up ball and approaches mother)
Mother: That's right. Get the ball. Get it.
                    (Gleason, 1977: 202)

In the first example, the mother expanded on her previous utterance; in the second, she verbalized the child's action. Her verbalization might function as would internal speech, which the child has not yet developed. It is important to understand that these repetitions are the mother's way of providing her own feedback to what her child does. This is how a mother shows that she has understood her child and that she accepts him or her as a speaking subject in their 'conversation'. Such feedback is vital, for it gives children the satisfaction of knowing that they are understood.

Messer believes that by repeating herself within a single verbal episode, a mother lets her child choose from among several equivalent utterances and adopt those that are easiest for him or her to interpret and understand. From this angle — child comprehension of maternal speech — the function of repetition perhaps changes depending on the child's age: at first it serves to acquaint children with labeling, and only later leads them to discover syntactic relationships.

In any case, these various discursive devices seem to arise out of a mother's concern with understanding her child and being understood by him or her.

We have now examined all of the features of this special child-directed speech register. Before we move on, two additional points should be made: this particular register is not used exclusively by mothers, nor is it the only register that mothers ever use when speaking to their child.

Shatz and Gelman (1977) have shown that as early as three years old, children know how to change their speech register when talking to very young children. They use the same devices that mothers do: heavy repetition, shorter utterances and attention getting. This register seems to go hand in hand with sociolinguistic sensitivities that children are believed to develop as they acquire all of their various communication skills.

In a comparative study between mothers and 'non-mothers' — young women having little experience with children — Snow (1972) showed that when the non-mothers had to talk to a child they assumed a register exactly like that of experienced mothers. Similar research focusing on fathers and other male adults has revealed that men also adopt a particular speech register resembling that of mothers.

In other words, everyone who truly wants to communicate with a child resorts to this same register: it is not exclusively maternal even though mothers may have their own special ways of formulating it. Comparative studies by J. A. Rondal (1980) have shown that while there are differences between maternal and paternal speech, both belong to the same register and fall within the parameters that we have described.

Besides not belonging to mothers alone, this speech register is not the only register that mothers use with their children. The great attention given to this speech mode can cause us to forget that there exists a completely different kind of speech that mothers use with their child. One of the mothers interviewed by Garnica described this other speech mode — perhaps unintentionally — when asked how she talked to her child: 'There are plenty of times I don't stop to think that he's two and I'll just mumble something at him or make some kind of demand on him and don't really think about whether or not he can understand it. And that's when he's most likely not to respond at all' (Garnica, 1977: 87). In the context of the interview, Garnica interpreted this remark as an expression of the concern that mothers have for establishing effective communication — the mother was aware of the fact that when she let herself go and did not think about her child's response, the child did not respond. But her remark also clearly refers to a dimension of speech that has been identified by Diatkine as 'free-flowing speech' (*le discours lâche*) (Diatkine, 1975b).

Maternal speech is also 'free-flowing'. Whereas mothers know how to offer their child 'quality' moments of verbal communication in a very special register, they also sometimes talk on and on to their baby without really trying to communicate with him or her at all, as Garnica's interviewee acknowledged. During such times, mothers no longer experience their child as a distinct subject but as an extension of themselves: they aren't talking to their child to tell him or her anything in particular or to establish communication on the child's level; they are simply talking 'about anything and everything' in the presence of their child. If a mother becomes aware of carrying on in this way, she will likely pass it off as insignificant or even silly.

However, as Diatkine (1976) points out, these words, spoken for no reason at all, are far from insignificant:

> Adults can let go more easily when caught between an illusion of commu-
> nication and the knowledge that their interlocutor does not understand:
> what they say 'doesn't matter'. Moreover, the one being spoken to consti-
> tutes an important part of the one speaking. The more adults believe that
> what they say is unimportant and the more they are generally unaware that
> it might mean something, the greater will be their abandon to fancy.
> (Diatkine, 1976: 602)

Diatkine sees this situation as a real 'state of grace' in which a mother can let herself regress with her child and not really be concerned about whether she and her child form a whole or two separate entities.

In sum, children experience a very complex sort of 'language immersion' that flows from their mother's relationship to them — a relationship of otherness and fusion. Out of this relationship emerge two complementary types of speech: *the special register* and *free-flowing speech*. This kind of language immersion is entirely different from the flow of words that might spill over children from television or radio, for those words are not specifically directed at them in the well-defined modalities we have described.

A mother who knows how to let her speech flow freely with her child is a mother who also knows how to talk to her child in a special speech register that is appropriately adapted to his or her abilities. Immersed in all this language, children eventually take to speaking themselves. Let's take a look at how this happens in each of these two modalities.

The effects of maternal speech on child language acquisition

Now that we have observed the unique way in which mothers talk to their young children, we should ask ourselves what the implications of this behavior are on children's language development. Roger Brown (1977) emphasizes that this is not the same as asking what a mother intends. Mothers might act with certain purposes in mind, but their actions can have effects that they never imagined. This distinction will become clear as we examine both types of maternal speech: the special speech register and free-flowing speech.

Effects of the special speech register

Whereas the mothers interviewed by Garnica (1977) realized that they made changes in register in order to communicate as effectively as possible, those whom Ferguson questioned about their verbal behavior with their child (1977) indicated that they were concerned about 'teaching their child language'. These are not conflicting responses. Brown notes that in the first case the mothers had been interviewed immediately after a taping session of them interacting with their child. In the second case they had been interviewed in an unrelated situation, outside of any mother–child exchange. Brown believes that the parents in this second group probably intellectualized their behavior somewhat and in so doing inflated their teaching intents. There are two reasons why teaching hardly seems to be parents' real and primary motivation.

First, young children also use this special register when they address those younger than themselves, yet they surely have not achieved the 'metalinguistic distance' from their own language that they would need to be able to 'teach' it. Children do, however, know how to 'get their message across' and make themselves understood in whatever situation they might find themselves, including having to adapt to the conversational constraints imposed by a baby interlocutor. In so doing they exhibit their desire to communicate, not to teach.

Second, the kind of simplification that occurs in the register mothers use hardly reveals a primary concern for teaching. As we have seen, maternal utterances might be brief but they are full of complex syntax. Rather than starting with the simplest structures and moving to the more complex as would a teacher, mothers offer their child a whole variety of structures all at once. In fact their approach offers not a single example of a simple-to-complex progression in syntax.

But this point raises an important question: is our definition of simplicity the same as children's? In her experiments on how children learn to read, Emilia Ferreiro (1979: 70) discovered that our definitions can diverge quite significantly from those of children: 'Children have their own definitions of "simple" and "hard" that for the most part do not coincide with our own'. (Ferreiro, 1979: 70)

Children might find their mother's use of complex syntax 'simple'. Gelman and Shatz (1977) found that mothers produce complex utterances specifically when guiding their child's actions or eliciting a response that they know the child is capable of. For example: '*Do you know what that is*? (said while the child was picking up a boat; child answered mother with "Um...boat")' (Gelman and Shatz, 1977: 53). Mothers reserve complex sentences of this type for situations in which the child can't help but understand given the context of the utterance.

Through context, mothers let their child *see* what is to be *understood*, thereby making their words clear and 'easy' for their child to understand despite their syntactic complexity. Basically a mother tries to *communicate;* this is her primary intention. Perhaps it is this very attitude that helps a mother discover what is 'simple' for her child in the language acquisition process. Without realizing it, she becomes a perfect teacher. She knows how to connect her utterances to the context in order to make them simple for the child to understand regardless of their syntactic structure.

In other words, it is simply by *communicating* that a mother guides her child into langauge, offering him or her what Snow (1972: 561) calls 'language lessons'. In these 'lessons' we find the same spirit of fun and enjoyment that we discovered in mother–infant preverbal dialogue. Here again it is the combination of *teaching* and *pleasure* that brings children to speak.

In a review of the research thus far conducted on this special speech register, Brown (1977) contends that no child learns to speak without the benefit of some of the features this register offers. In conclusion he states that he now has

an answer to a parental question for which I have never had an answer. The question, of course, is 'How can a concerned mother facilitate her child's learning of language?' My answer [...] is: 'Believe that your child can understand more than he or she can say, and seek, above all, to communicate. To understand and be understood [...] There is no set of rules of how to talk to a child that can even approach what you unconsciously know. If you concentrate on communicating, everything else will follow' (Brown, 1977: 26).

In sum, mothers use this 'special speech register' in order to communicate, which is precisely why what they offer their child constitutes true language instruction. Yet Brown recognizes that not all children have equal opportunity to enjoy the benefits of this special speech register, as has been made clear in comparative studies aimed at showing the ways in which this register fosters language acquisition in children.

Research by Robert Hess and Virginia Shipman (1965) reveals that poor language nourishment — nourishment inadequately suited to a child's abilities — can actually hinder that child's language development.

Keith Nelson, Gaye Carskaddon and John Bonvillian (1973) have also shown that *quality of conversation* is the most significant variable in language acquisition. Diatkine expresses this same opinion when he says, 'Perhaps children in privileged circles speak well not so much because they are spoken to in proper language but because they are *spoken* to!' (Diatkine *et al.*, 1977: 123).

These findings corroborate research conducted by Gordon Wells (1978) on factors that contribute to healthy language development:

Of all the variables describing the linguistic environment of the child, it was the range of Pragmatic Functions in the speech addressed to the child that was the best predictor of the child's language development — both of his command of the system and of the range of functions for which he used it. (Wells, 1978: 466–7)

Such are the effects of the adapted speech register. Now let's take a look at the effects of free-flowing speech.

The effects of free-flowing speech

Mothers don't appear to be trying to accomplish anything in particular *vis-à-vis* their child when they let themselves ramble on in the baby's presence, not really trying to communicate or establish an interaction. Yet this behavior seems to have quite an impact on children's ability to learn language. For it is in this context that many affects pass between mother and child, the child often echoing what the mother says. This is also how children acquire pat expressions — including ones their parents would prefer them not to know! Parents often wonder where their child could have possibly picked up this 'four-letter word' or that 'adult' expression. It would appear that children glean them from free-flowing speech. Tatiana Slama-Cazacu (1977) notes that when children 'echo' adult speech they use highly developed 'syntax blocks' made up of complex elements that they don't know how to use other than in these fixed expressions.

So one function of free-flowing speech seems to be that it allows children to pick up on speech despite their lack of linguistic baggage. Yet the primary significance of free-flowing speech is to be found at a much deeper level of linguistic interaction. We know that communication always involves an intimate connection between making contact and transmitting information. The varying importance of each function relative to the other is what creates the full spectrum of possible types of exchange.

The difference between 'free-flowing speech' and the 'special register' can be explained in terms of this spectrum. Free-flowing speech is intended almost exclusively for the purpose of making contact. A mother rambles on simply because her child is there and because he or she counts in her eyes — the child is the catalyst of her speech. This results in an exceptional kind of contact. As we have seen, the mother does not have to choose between seeing her child as an extension of herself or as a distinct person. The atmosphere that envelops free-flowing speech is reminiscent of what was said earlier about transitional objects: it creates an aura in which no distinction between the subjective and objective world and no 'awesome' decision has to be made. Our need to resolve these distinctions and decisions as painlessly as possible is in fact the guiding force behind our psychical lives.

It is quite probably the texture of free-flowing speech that allows children to gain from speech that is specially adapted to them and sets apart the subjective from the objective. Children are able to become interlocutors in this special register because, parallel to such exchanges, there are times when their mother lets her speech flow freely and exempts either of them from having to assume a position — her words are spoken for no reason but the mere pleasure of it.

So each of these two exchange modalities — free-flowing and adapted speech — fulfills an important function; each has meaning only in relation to the other. In fact, free-flowing speech appears to create a transitional space in which adapted speech can be understood and actually 'teach' the child to speak. With this in mind, we shall now observe how a child's first words emerge.

A child's first words

In the preverbal period children establish themselves as speaking subjects. They 'talk' insofar as they manipulate both the illocutionary and locutionary aspects of language. They make speech acts in their own way and know how to take their place in a dialogue, express requests, orders, affirmations and so on. Furthermore, these expressions mark the beginnings of reference and predication as children use them to signify the content of their 'speech'.

Children thus engage in sophisticated *linguistic* activity before they ever speak. Even at this early stage they already communicate in a verbal modality and know the basics of how such communication works. Already they understand some of what is said directly to them and even some of that which is not. This means that they have managed to set up a whole range of signifiers and to construct a system of distinctions within their little world. Yet they don't talk. What more has to happen before they do?

From speaking subject to naming subject

Children accompany all of their preverbal 'speech' with vocalizations, but these sounds cannot be considered 'words'. On this point everyone agrees.

Children might make sounds, like 'Mmm' or 'na-na', that have specific illocutionary value — for example they could serve to make a request. In very specific and ritualized contexts children also might make 'semi-referential' vocalizations. For example, in a game of give-and-take with an object, children might always produce the same sound to mean that it is their turn. Or again, children might use something like 'ma-ma-ma' (one of the sounds that mothers strongly reinforce) to refer to their mother yet indiscriminately use it to designate other people as well.

Even though all of these vocalizations are easily interpreted, none qualifies as a 'word', for none can be said to have a specific and fixed referent. This is probably the criterion we all apply to tell if the sounds children make are really words or not. We know that even though a sound like 'papa' might closely resemble one of our own words, it doesn't really qualify as a word unless it always refers back to a particular referent. On the other hand, once we hear a particular sound being used for a fixed referent, we know that it is a word even if it is unlike any we've ever heard. As a matter of fact, the first word children utter is often of their own creation.

In what specific circumstances do those first words form? As an answer to this question, we will present Michèle Perron-Borelli's (1976) detailed observation of how her daughter, Catherine, came to speak her first word at 14 months old.

That morning Catherine had been on a long and eventful outing with her mother and had to deal with new faces in new places. As if this weren't hard enough, Catherine encountered a very disconcerting problem: in the new place where she had been taken, she couldn't even walk by herself because the floor had just been waxed and she slipped with every step.

For Catherine, this was '*a minima*, a traumatic situation' (ibid.: 688). She was experiencing two types of loss: loss of a good and unfailing mother who now made her go through all this torment, and loss of her recently acquired ability to walk by herself. Catherine was simultaneously experiencing object loss and narcissistic loss.

Mother and daughter then went to Catherine's grandmother's house. Finding herself in a familiar framework, Catherine relaxed. That's when her mother took a teddy bear out of her sack. This teddy bear was one of Catherine's favorite toys, one that she had claimed as a transitional object — an object halfway between objective and subjective reality.

When Catherine saw her teddy bear she took it in a frenzy. Her mother explains:

> She grabbed it out of my hands, almost violently and she held it close crying out 'yne-yne' [ɲə–ɲɔ]. She repeated 'yne-yne' several times, holding the teddy bear out so she could see it, then hugging it close again. I immediately noticed something different about this word 'yne-yne'. The distinctness with which it was spoken set it apart from her usual vocalizations. The overall scene and the fact that she kept repeating this word made its significant association with the teddy bear clear. (ibid.: 682)

Just getting her teddy bear back was not enough for Catherine. She felt the need to 'name' it and thereby affirm its unique existence as a 'good object' like her mother during pleasant moments. In naming her teddy bear, Catherine in fact used one of the sounds that she would make during tender moments with her mother.

Thus 'named', the teddy bear's status as a transitional object changed to that of a real object on which Catherine projected the image of the good mother who hadn't been there for her throughout that troubling morning. But Catherine was able to make this projection only because she had succeeded in internalizing this good mother through the experience of on-going positive communication with her.

Whereas the teddy bear became Catherine's mother, it also became Catherine herself: through this repairing process that Catherine set up, she passed from a 'having' level to a 'being' level. In order to deal with her object loss, she internalized her mother to become her. In the process of restoring herself, Catherine also entered into her own personal existence.

When it was nap time and her mother was about to leave her alone, Catherine very distinctly said 'yne-yne'. Her mother understood that her daughter wanted her teddy bear and went to get it. This was an intense experience for both mother and daughter: Catherine 'was able to confirm that stating the signifier was enough to make the missing object reappear' (ibid.: 690), and her mother was left in awe by the 'miracle of communication' (ibid.: 690). Catherine's mother had certainly been communicating with her daughter all along, but this was the first time that their communication had been so 'obvious' (ibid.: 690).

Through her act of denomination, Catherine took on her full stature as a subject *vis-à-vis* her mother: she had broken out of the insular world of a dyadic relationship and dealt with the trauma of separation. Here we see the beginnings of a clearly triangular relationship: 'The mother to whom the linguistic message is directed is no longer the exclusive object of her child's desire; she is able to understand and respond to this message because she herself is willing to relinquish this exclusivity' (ibid.: 690).

By sharing meaning, semantic content and the expression 'yne-yne', mother and daughter were brought into a new relationship in which they each defined themselves in terms of an acknowledged 'it', This was a significant change that affected both of them deeply. The 'first-word' experience is a very meaningful one that significantly expands both mother and child into 'something more.' It represents a huge leap in 'becoming' and in recognizing each other as subjects.

On the train ride home Catherine, who had been given the teddy bear by her mother, put it carefully back in the sack 'with all the gestures of maternal care, as though to protect it or help it go to sleep. It was perfectly clear that she had resolutely and competently undertaken to care for her teddy bear on this trip...' (ibid.: 683). Looking at the closed sack that contained her teddy bear, Catherine said 'yne-yne', not to ask her mother for or about it, but to confirm and be reassured that it was still there. Labeling brings back what is unseen or absent and gives one solace in the process.

Carefully attending to her teddy bear was clearly Catherine's way of lavishing on herself all the care she had been deprived of throughout the morning's trip. Through her actions she was internalizing her mother and thereby identifying with her. This is not mere imitation, but 'a distancing imitation' (Doumic-Girard, 1980: 505) that makes it possible to internalize someone else. Through this relationship with her teddy bear, Catherine thus achieved a certain degree of objectivity: she became both a 'me' (her internalized mother) and an 'observed me' (her teddy bear). The next morning, earnestly searching her mother's face, Catherine used the expression 'yne-yne' for a different stuffed bear that was up on a shelf out of her reach. Her mother 'immediately understood her request on two different levels: as a practical request (to give her the bear that she couldn't reach herself) and as a symbolic request (to confirm the value of her semantic generalization)' (Perron-Borelli, 1976: 683).

The labeling process thus allowed Catherine to make a generalization: she grouped together new objects that could be *equivalent* to the mother–object but which were *distinct* from it. This is the point at which Catherine began entering speech as an active speaker. In the following days she showed a high degree of originality and creativity in her use of new words.

Having retraced each step that Catherine took in beginning to name things, we can see that this passage from a speaking subject to a naming subject grounds children in a new relationship with the world and with others. Once children are able to differentiate themselves from their mother they can identify with her. They establish themselves more deeply as subjects and become capable of maintaining an objective connection with reality. This is what enables children to enter into a triangular relationship.

Once children share common semantic content used by others, they can begin to communicate linguistically with other people. Even though children often continue to communicate primarily with their mother, their newfound speech allows them to carry on verbal exchanges with all of the members of their family. This is very important for their personal development: through language children are able to achieve multiple identifications.

As Catherine's case clearly shows, children utter their 'first word' for the primary purpose of naming something in order to stave off anxieties that arise from various kinds of loss — object loss and narcissistic loss. Only secondarily do these names serve as illocutionary acts such as making a request, an order, etc. — children already have multiple preverbal means for accomplishing these acts.

Many of us have observed how much children delight in naming for naming's sake when they are first beginning to talk. Labeling does in fact play a very important role in children's acquisition of speech: it offers them a mental framework for dealing with states of loss that would otherwise become quickly unbearable. For children, write Diatkine *et al.* (1977: 119), words are a way of 'not succumbing to the pain of desire and transforming that pain into pleasure'. These striking words powerfully express the ordeal children go through on their path to speech acquisition. This process becomes unbearable and cannot be satisfactorily accomplished unless children apply a good deal of their language activity to play, 'where distinctions between object and desire, and between narcissism and the objective world in effect don't exist. These are the times when children ramble on to themselves, talking just to talk' (ibid.: 119). This is how Diatkine explains children's need for 'speech that says nothing' (ibid.: 119), which we will now examine.

The need for speech that says nothing

When children begin to name things and to speak, they don't drop the vocalizations that they produced in preverbal activity. Lallation does not stop when talking starts; it continues and remains valuable to children as a transitional device by which they can remove themselves from the 'awesome' dilemma of presence and absence.

Lallations help children handle being alone when their mother is absent; these sounds comfort them as does their mother's presence. They also enable children to be alone even when their mother is present. In other words, it lets them become self-initiating even in her presence. This is the situation in which children truly develop a capacity for being alone.

Echolalic repetition also belongs to this kind of transitional activity, as do all the word games in which children indulge. Children speak for the pleasure of sounds, sounds that bring them back to language as they first knew it — an ever-present background of sound and speech full of rhythm, color and melody. This continuum is what eventually enables children to distinguish words and phrases, their skill largely depending on how rich it has been.

The custom of telling nursery and counting rhymes to children exists in all language communities and responds to children's thirst for spoken sounds. It is often said that children are poets. Whether or not this adage holds true, we do know that children are fascinated with stories, poems, and tales. Even though the content may be over their heads, they listen, utterly absorbed, and will beg to have a particular story or poem repeated again and again, word for word. This need continues in children for a long time, even after they have begun to use speech 'seriously'.

Concerning serious uses of speech, we must remember that a child's first labels are quickly followed by short two-word sentences like 'mean dog' or 'baby sleep'. 'At a very young age, children realize that in verbal communication, meaning can consist not just of one, but of a group of words', argues Miguel Siguan Soler (1977: 66). Once children reach the naming stage, they immediately apply to speech the predication techniques they learned in preverbal communication.

But children certainly don't use speech just for saying 'serious' words and forming well predicated sentences. They devote much of their verbal activity to sound games in which they leave behind any concern for content and manipulate words — even whole sentences — just for the pleasure of their consonance.

Ruth Weir became very interested in this type of verbal activity in her son. Here is an example of the kind of thing he would say before falling asleep at two and a half years old:

go for glasses
go for them
go to the top
go throw
go for blouse
pants
go for shoes.
(Weir, 1970: 115)

Observing the same sorts of verbal games in children, McNeill (1970) notes that they sometimes resemble a fugue:

Adult: That's the tattooed man.
Child: Tooman. Tattoo man. Find too tattoo man. Tattoo man. Who dat? Tattoo. Too man go, mommy? Tooman. Tattoo man go? Who dat? Read dat. Tractor dere. Tattoo man.
(McNeill, 1970: 107)

Diatkine attributes a very important function to this type of utterance: children develop their ability to say things by exercising their ability to say nothing. We see in children what we saw in mothers: a need for two kinds of speech, 'serious' speech to say things and 'free-flowing' speech to say nothing. We must point out, however, that children don't use this second kind of speech only for 'saying nothing'. It also expresses their need to return to their first experience of language as a place of enrapturing sounds. Here, language becomes a game again, a game that eases children into the 'awesome' dialectic of speech meant to 'say' something.

This ability to talk to say nothing is fundamental to the language acquisition process in children — a fact that 'serious' adults too often forget. Diatkine finds it deplorable that some parents and many teachers so fully ignore this side of speech — speech spoken purely for the pleasure of it. He emphasizes the importance of mothers humoring their child's nonsensical speech and joining in the enjoyment of verbal games rather than trying to give sense to nonsense; for 'children learn to talk by playing with words' (Diatkine, 1976: 600). Moreover, such games are an 'essential prerequisite for schooling' (ibid.: 604). Children must, for example, be able to reconcile reading 'it's raining' on the blackboard when it's sunny outside. What is asked of children at school presupposes that they can become interested in a 'meaningless language offered by a meaningless person' (Diatkine *et al.*, 1977: 120). As we will see, recognizing that children must be able to say things that do not mean much to them will have very specific pedagogical implications when it comes to educating deaf children.

Summary: Children acquire speech by communicating

To illustrate how the scientific approach to language acquisition has evolved, Gleason (1977) explains:

Sitting in peoples' homes listening to them say to their young children things like 'Where's the ball? There's the ball. Give Mommy the ball. That's right, give me the ball. Give it to me.' hardly seems an activity that might lead to changes in theoretical models of language development, yet it has done just that. (Gleason, 1977: 199)

While linguists still recognize the essential role of neurological development in the language acquisition process, they have recently begun to acknowledge the importance of *communication*. Language learning particularly depends on the genuine contact that a child has known through being addressed by older individuals. Such contact usually includes elements of the outside world: it is a process between two partners with an implied third dimension, namely the context in which the exchange takes place.

This new perspective on how children acquire speech solved the dilemma of having to choose between two conflicting theories of language acquisition — both of which grew out of information theory, with its excessive focus on codes and syntactic models. According to Bruner (1978: 203), we were caught between an 'impossible' theory based on a doctrine of association that would never reveal how children begin to talk, and a 'magical' theory based on some innate predisposition to language — which doesn't explain the 'how' of language acquisition either.

If we simply observe how mothers talk to their young children we can move beyond these contradictory theories. Primarily concerned with responding to their child's need to communicate, mothers know how to adapt their speech to fit their child's abilities perfectly. Children do not learn speech from a corpus of usually non-grammatical, incomplete and hardly intelligible sentences, as those who theorized about innate language acquisition assumed. Quite to the contrary, mothers use clear, easily understood speech and draw heavily on the communication situation in order to achieve the exchange, for they want to be understood by their child. In other words, they use context to get their message across. This is why children manage to understand what they couldn't begin to decode. Mothers adapt their speech most notably when it comes to using language for pragmatic and discursive purposes, in a sense bringing their children to *hear with their eyes*. The visual channel is as important (if not more so) than the auditory. According to Macnamara (1972), children are able to learn to speak because they can deduce the meaning of what they hear from what they see. What they see is the *context* of the exchange and all of the *extra-verbal communication* provided by mimicry, facial expressions, eye contact, expressive gestures and body posture.

Furthermore, mothers use their child's own extra-verbal activity as the basis for conversation. They first seek to understand and interpret these cues and then respond to them. The mother's behavior relies heavily on that of her child, who really is an active partner in the exchange.

Children are caught up in verbal communication right from birth. We have talked about preverbal communication as preceding verbal communication, but never is communication solely preverbal. *Expressively*, children go through a preverbal period, but *receptively* they soak up their mother's verbal attention right from the day they are born. And conversely, children don't simply lose their many preverbal abilities once they begin to acquire verbal skills. They continue to employ a rich array of channels in order to transmit and receive messages and establish dialogue.

Preoccupied as we are with verbal interaction, we tend to forget that these exchanges occur only within an elaborate framework of extra-verbal communication. Eye-gaze, facial expressions, gestures and posture are inextricably linked to each and every one of our spoken utterances. Since this kind of extra-verbal communication precedes speech in children, it is labelled 'preverbal communication' — despite the fact that nothing verbal is ever said without it.

Speech contributes to a process of *total communication* that includes all verbal and extra-verbal communication. We prefer the term *extra-verbal* to *nonverbal*, for the latter is a negative definition that connotes opposition. Such labeling only reinforces the emphasis put on verbal communication, as if it could stand alone. *Extra-verbal*, however, defines this kind of communication not by what it is not, but by what it is: communication that exceeds the framework of language but without which language could not exist. There is no contradiction or break between these two types of communication: as conceptualized in Figure 2.1, they are related conjunctively, not disjunctively.

Bruner's observation that linguistic schemata develop during preverbal communication only reaffirms the conjunctive relationship between verbal and extra-verbal communication. Emphasizing the importance of extra-verbal

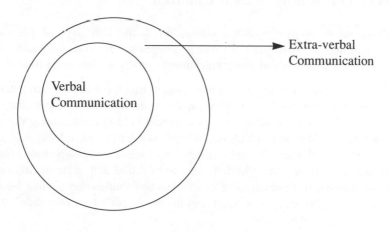

Verbal Communication

Extra-verbal Communication

FIGURE 2.1

communication, Margaret Bullowa (1979) goes so far as to ask, 'Why should language be the prototype for all human communication, a great deal of which is extra-lingual, even among adults?' (Bullowa, 1979: 15).

Whereas communication is what enables children to acquire speech, speech in turn expands their opportunities for communication. Children use speech — labeling in particular — as a prime means of making distinctions as they go about situating themselves in relation to their mother and the world around them. In and through their own speech, children become subjects able to deal with separation and enter into a more objective relationship with reality. Communication then tends to take on its fullness as an exchange among distinct individuals who, having recognized themselves as such, also acknowledge each other's unique existence.

Children don't use this identity-forming speech solely for communication: they also play with words and sounds for the mere pleasure of it. Playing with language is an important ingredient in speech acquisition. What was necessary for preverbal communication is also necessary for verbal communication: an atmosphere of fun and pleasure. Without it, there can be no communication and, consequently, no speech.

Throughout this chapter we have been looking at how children acquire speech. Now, in our concluding discussion, we will consider what these observations imply when it comes to educating deaf children.

Conclusion: The Speech Ability of All Children and How to Preserve This Ability in Deaf Children

Observations of mother–infant interaction in the first days of life have revealed that human young are born with a competence for communicating and that they need interaction and communication as vitally as they need food.

Not even a half a century ago, it was thought that it could be detrimental to show babies affection: holding, rocking and otherwise stimulating them could be harmful. These attitudes resulted from the widely held opinion among doctors and nurses in the 1900s that 'indulging' infants was dangerous. Educational philosophy, heavily influenced by behaviorism, only reinforced the pediatric theories and practices of the time. Children were to be raised with regimentation and in cold objectivity. In describing the predicament of mothers up against 'scientific' authorities who often knew much less than they, but whom they didn't dare disobey, Montagu (1971) writes:

> ...And so millions of mothers sat and cried along with their babies, but, as genuinely loving mothers obedient to the best thinking on the subject, bravely resisted the 'animal instinct' to pick them up and comfort them in their arms. Most mothers felt that this could not be right, but who were they to argue with the authorities? (Montagu, 1971: 126)

Today, mothers of deaf children find themselves in a similar situation — only amplified — in the face of experts whose advice often clashes with their own intuitions.

Once scientists recognized the infant's capacity for interacting with its mother (something that mothers knew all along), new perspectives opened up in the field of language acquisition. Now linguists are not interested only in what children say once they have started talking; they look at the overall behavior of these little beings seeking to communicate — something they do before they ever speak.

Children use multiple channels to understand and be understood. To use sociolinguist Dell Hymes' (1972) expression, they develop 'communicative competence' well before they talk.

Thus, language is now studied and understood as being part of the exchange process that characterizes children's interaction with those around them. Every aspect of children's cognitive, social and language development begins with interaction. Communication competence is what joins these aspects together. By the sixth month, a dialogue develops between mother and infant in which the infant can assume an *active* role. Through dialogue, children begin to master all sorts of 'perceptive, motor, conceptual, social and linguistic' skills, contends Bruner (1975: 256), who has shown that children discover the elemental techniques of dialogue, reference and predication in none other than these early exchanges.

In other words, *communication* competence leads to *linguistic* competence. A child's language history begins at birth and depends on all of those first mother–infant interactions and on the mother's own anticipation of her little-one's communication abilities. Not surprisingly, each child's history is unique, and enormous speech differences exist among everyday three to four-year-old children.

Mothers accompany their first preverbal interactions with speech. Insofar as a mother addresses her child as a little being seeking to communicate, she can't help but talk — for her, speech is communication *par excellence*.

In a healthy development of such exchanges, a mother welcomes everything that her child does as something he or she 'wants' to tell her, and she then responds in an appropriate way, drawing her child into a meaningful dialogue relationship.

Just like any other child, deaf children seem to benefit fully from these early exchanges, developing their linguistic abilities through ritualized games and activities that are based on shared attention. Although the sounds of their mother's voice cannot reach them, they do perceive everything that envelops her speech: the look in her eye, the expressions on her face, her gestures, her body movements. We have already shown how important the visual channel is to these first interactions: children are able to understand them by relying on extra-verbal communication. At this stage, speech depends entirely on context.

Even though deaf children don't hear what their mother says, they are able to take full advantage of their joint interactions. Here we would agree with Asa Hammar's (1980) assertion that 'as vision plays such an important role in the interaction during the first year, *the deaf child is not really handicapped at this age of life*'[6] (Hammar, 1980: 6). Blind children, on the other hand, do suffer a real handicap when it comes to entering into these early interactions that depend so heavily on sight.

But the deaf child's language history can get off to a perfectly good start.

In the first year of life deaf children acquire a solid core of linguistic skills. During this period they enjoy a healthy relationship with their mother and establish themselves as *speaking* subjects. How can these skills be preserved?

At the beginning of the second year, communication starts to depend more on the auditory channel and mothers rely less on context when they speak. At this point communication thus becomes more difficult for deaf children.

Whereas their whole behavior seems to announce the imminence of speech, those first words never come. This is when deafness is most often first suspected, usually by the child's mother. The discovery of deafness almost irreparably breaks off the interaction that existed between them. As Elizabeth Wilson, mother of a deaf child, explains:

> Before my child was diagnosed as deaf, I seemed to be more in tune with his behavior *as a way of telling me something*.[7] We respond to a baby's behavior without much trouble. We know a hungry cry, a sleepy cry, a wet-diaper cry. The child indicates a need and we respond. Somehow when my child was diagnosed as deaf, I stopped seeing him as a child and looked at him as DEAF. (Wilson, 1975: 29)

Here Wilson clearly describes the break that occurred in her relationship with her son when she discovered that he was deaf. She no longer saw him as a subject communicating in his own way as she always had before. Seeing him as deaf meant that she lost her ability to communicate with him at all because she thought that being deaf equaled being mute, that is, incapable of 'saying' anything.

The emphasis she placed on verbal communication caused her to ignore all the extra-verbal communication that envelops speech. Before the handicap was discovered, Wilson and her son had shared a lot of information and interaction through *extra-verbal* communication alone.

When deafness was diagnosed, both mother and child thus found their communication severely disturbed. Because she placed primary importance on speech that her child couldn't hear, Wilson lost her ability to interact with him in a different mode as she had always unknowingly done when, unaware of his deafness, she had talked to him naturally. Meanwhile, her son lost the atmosphere of dialogue and the framework of meaning that had upheld all of his interactions with his mother.

If this rupture lasts for long it can seriously affect the deaf child's communicative and linguistic abilities.

As Wilson explains, she changed her behavior upon realizing what a break in communication her attitude had imposed on her child when his deafness was discovered: 'I was encouraged to do this [only think of her child as deaf] by the information I got... Somehow we parents put aside our intuition and instincts, maybe because we feel inferior because we don't have a degree or special training' (we all know that specialists tend to emphasize speech above all else in the communication process) 'but we have a responsibility to follow our instincts. At the same time, members of the medical and educational professions have a unique opportunity to learn from us and to support our understanding'. And what does Wilson understand? 'We must learn to communicate [with our deaf child] on his terms and to understand his behaviors as communication' (Wilson, 1975: 29).

As a mother, Wilson thus discovered how to act with her deaf child as she always had, letting her child's behavior define her own according to that wonderful pedagogy that mothers practice without even realizing it.

Her deaf child is first and foremost a child. Though he happens to be deaf, he remains a full-fledged speaking subject, a being of communication and language. Wilson will continue to seek to dialogue and communicate with her son just as every mother does with her child. As we have seen, mothers who accept their child as a partner know how to adapt their speech to their child's abilities by developing a *multisensory* web of meaning.

Chapter 1 led us to the conclusion that deaf children can't be considered but as speaking subjects. In Chapter 2 we now discover that deaf children, like all children, develop a real competence for communication and language through early preverbal exchanges with their mother. The only way to safeguard these abilities is to continue to treat deaf children like complete speaking subjects after their deafness has been discovered. Even though they are deaf, these children need to live in communication with others and participate in meaningful exchanges — exchanges in which their way of expressing themselves is recognized and responded to in an appropriate way.

Deaf children experience all of the same needs that other children do: they too need speech that is adapted to their abilities. How can this be given to them? To answer this question, we must first define what constitutes a mother tongue.

Notes to Chapter 2

1. In this and the following chapter we use the term 'mother' to mean the child's primary caretaker.
2. The mother provides feedback in the sense that she confirms what her child 'said', while offering a correct label.
3. Congress Proceedings, *Developing Home Training Programs for Hearing Impaired Children*. Albuquerque, New Mexico, 1976.
4. Ibid.
5. By repetition we mean not only *literal* repetition but also *semantic* repetition, that is, a mother's successive statements showing little change in content.
6. Emphasis added.
7. Emphasis added.

3 Toward a Definition of Mother Tongue: The Mother's Role in Child Language Acquisition

It might seem odd that we would propose to define something as obvious as *mother tongue*. According to the dictionary, it is 'the language of one's mother; the language naturally acquired in infancy and childhood; one's first language' (Websters, 1976). Who would disagree?

Yet isn't this *mother tongue* usually the language spoken by the child's father and siblings as well? Furthermore, most families speak the language of the country in which they live, so doesn't *mother tongue* actually mean the 'national language' of the country of which the child is a citizen?

The expression *mother tongue* connects the notion of *tongue*, or language, to that of *mother* — and somehow this connection seems justified. Here we will examine why. In Chapter 2 we noted that the special speech register mothers use to talk to their child does not belong to them alone. Everyone uses it to talk to any child who does not yet know how to speak as grown-ups do.

Yet mothers do seem to play a special role in their child's appropriation of language. In order to observe and define this role, we must go back to the first year of life, that year when children can survive only in intimate contact with their mother. During such contact a mother draws her child into preverbal dialogue which is usually accompanied by verbal conversation on her part. Very early, the child's participation in these interactions becomes intentional and reciprocal.

Maternal behavior is unique when it comes to forming this nucleus of communicative and linguistic abilities: a mother not only seeks to understand what her child 'means' to tell her, she also actively shares in each of her child's 'statements', be it a look, an expressive face, a smile, a vocalization or a gesture. A mother clues in to her child's language, to her child's way of expressing him or herself, and then responds appropriately in her own words.

M. A. K. Halliday (1979) closely observed such behavior by keeping a journal on how his son's 'protolanguage' developed from birth to 12 months. During a mother–infant interaction at six months he observed his child's first unmistakably 'meaningful act'. From this first meaningful act developed a whole 'little language' that the mother knew how to interpret each step of the way. As Halliday explains:

> This tracking of a child's language by his mother, and perhaps others, is a remarkable phenomenon that has been paid very little notice. It is something that takes place below the level of conscious awareness; those involved cannot, as a rule, describe what they are doing, and if the mother, for example, is asked what the child has been saying she is quite likely to contend that he wasn't saying anything at all — he can't talk yet. Of course he can't talk yet, in the mother tongue.[1] But he is talking in the child tongue; and the mother is responding all the time in a way which can be explained in no other way than as a response to language. (Halliday, 1979: 180)

'Before the mother tongue comes the child tongue', contends Halliday (ibid.: 172). This is an extremely important point that helps us zero in a bit further on what is so unique about the mother's role in child language acquisition. Only once a mother has received and acknowledged her *child's* language and given him or her the pleasure of being understood will she offer her child her own language: her language is a *response* to her child's. The *mother tongue*, then, is actually an *exchange* of 'languages'.

Mothers are accepting and attentive toward their baby without even always realizing it; this behavior certainly doesn't change when it comes to language. Although Halliday was looking at language, and Pawlby at imitation (see pp. 42–43), they both came to similar conclusions: mothers prepare their child to imitate them by first imitating their child; but they do so quite unknowingly and don't realize that they are the ones who set the example.

The same goes for language. The *mother tongue* is a bridge that a mother extends to her child. It's what enables children to cross over from their *own language* to the *language of others* — from being understood just by their mother to being understood by others as well. By allowing for an exchange of languages, the *mother tongue* breaks open the dual mother–infant relationship and propels children into a language understood and spoken by all.

Mothers may play an essential role in their child's acquisition of the language used around them, but this is not to say that fathers and others close to the child do not play an important part as well — quite to the contrary.

When we consider what a *mother tongue* actually is, we realize that children really do need a *privileged interlocutor* (usually the mother) in order to enter into speech, that is, the speech used by all those who encircle and take care of them.

As we have seen, mother–infant interactions in the first year of life set up a whole series of procedures that, in Bruner's (1975: 261) view, allow children to 'crack the linguistic code'. This breakthrough is made possible by an exchange of 'languages' between the child's 'speech' and the mother's.

Thus defined, *mother tongue* is a remarkable yet little appreciated phenomenon. Children's speech does not emerge out of a no-man's-land: it emerges out of the *mother tongue*, out of all that mother and infant share as they relate to each other and interact. Before children can go exploring other worlds and other interactions they need to inhabit this motherland where their own 'speech' is acknowledged. Unfortunately, many children seem to end up in kindergarten linguistically handicapped because they have been denied this motherland of a *mother tongue*.

The *mother tongue* phenomenon can thus be appreciated in negative terms as well. Gertrud Wyatt (1969), a child psychoanalyst who deals with the language difficulties many children exhibit, has pointed out that these problems are linked to a mother having been unable to provide her child with a 'verbal model'. Such mothers, unable to respond to their child's messages in the right way and at the right time, end up depriving the child of the pleasure of being understood. Wyatt's whole clinical approach emphasizes the importance of first receiving the child's speech so as to adapt one's own language to it. In her therapy sessions, Wyatt is able to achieve what some mothers accomplish spontaneously as they offer their child their language in exchange for the child's:

> We propose that all good teaching, or good therapy, requires two interrelated modes of communication. First, the adult, through listening and observation, must ascertain what information the child has already stored and understood and what skills he already commands; second, it must be the adult, the more developed organism, who consciously matches his style of communication with that of the child, the less developed one. (Wyatt, 1969: 14)

This therapy process closely resembles what occurs as children receive their *mother tongue* as defined above.

In her psychotherapy practice for young children with delayed language, Alice Doumic-Girard (Doumic-Girard *et al.*, 1975) also finds a clear correlation linking language delay to communication difficulties encountered in early mother–infant interactions. In such cases, the mother doesn't know how to 'talk' to her child, that is, how to integrate her language into extra-verbal communication that will satisfy her child's exchange needs. In discussing preverbal communication we described the multisensory environment that envelops the very beginnings of speech. In Doumic-Girard's experience, effective treatment hinges on just such multisensory communication.

Yet some mothers insulate themselves from the emotional involvement this total communication entails. Rather than 'talk' to their child, they 'teach' him or her to talk, sterilizing their communication by adopting an intellectual approach. These mothers lose their intuitive ability to understand the messages their child conveys, and consequently don't respond 'on par', that is, 'with a very special language that envelops words in a multisensory web of meaning' (Doumic-Girard *et al.*, 1975: 182).

In treating these linguistically delayed children Doumic-Girard has the mother join in the child's therapy sessions so that together they might make up for lost time in a communication-restoring atmosphere of induced regression. This helps the mother to better understand and respond to her child, and thereby establish a *mother tongue* that will introduce the child to the language spoken by others.

These observations of how children with language delays are treated make one thing clear: in the first year of a child's life, when the mother–infant relationship is so predominant, there comes a crucial moment — the moment when the mother is able to interpret her child's 'statement' and respond in 'her' language. In that moment the mother creates a bridge between the child's means of expression — which she, as the child's privileged partner, understands — and the way that those around the child generally express themselves through a commonly shared language.

In order to acquire language, children need to be accepted in their own way of expressing themselves, as different as it may be from the language spoken around them. In other words, children do not acquire commonly shared speech unless they have been received in their own.

Figure 3.1 visually represents what we have discussed in this chapter.

The *mother tongue* bridge means nothing without its two banks: the child's 'statements' on the one side and the mother's language (which is shared by others in the child's environment) on the other.

The *mother tongue* process does not insulate and 'ghettoize' mother and child: it actually propels children into the language used by those around them. Thus mothers do play a primary role in their child's acquisition of language during the first year of life. Incidentally, they also serve as interpreters between the

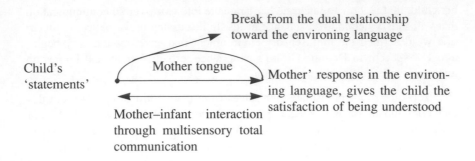

child and other family members, particularly the father, during this period when the child is not yet able to express him or herself in such a way as to be understood by all.

The *mother tongue* process thus builds a *communication bridge* between the child and others. Not only does this bridge give children access to the language used around them, it lets them be understood by others through the intermediary of their mother. Again, this all happens in the very first year of life in an atmosphere of pleasure and satisfaction.

Deaf children also need to go through this process of passing from two-way communication with their mother to wider communication with others. Just as any child, deaf infants need a *mother tongue*. But how can they be given one? Their lack of hearing has cut them off from the language spoken around them. What kind of bridge can connect these two worlds so painfully separated by deafness and create an exchange between the way deaf children express themselves and the way statements are made around them?

These are the questions we will be addressing in Part Two as we focus on the deaf child.

Note to Chapter 3

1.   Here Halliday uses 'mother tongue' in its widely recognized sense, not as we more narrowly define it in this chapter.

Part Two
The Deaf Child

In Part One we showed what speaking is and how children learn to talk. In Part Two we turn to deaf children. *Who are these children we call deaf?* Our approach of considering them in the reality of their lives, leads us to *Sign Language* and an understanding of how *deaf children acquire speech.* They too need a *mother tongue* in specific modalities that we will describe.

4 Who Are These Children We Call Deaf?

Hearing people have a very hard time imagining what it is like to be deaf. To those so dependent on their ability to hear, deafness seems like a strange, almost inconceivable world. The sense of sound shapes hearing people's whole way of living, speaking and communicating — which leads them to believe that the deaf live in a very empty world, and that many doors are shut to them.

Such attitudes inevitably have destructive repercussions on the lives of the deaf themselves. Seen only in terms of what they lack, the deaf suffer more from the way people act toward them than they do from their own deafness. In his book *A Deaf Adult Speaks Out*, Leo Jacobs (1980. 132) — a math teacher who was born deaf — writes about his years in school: 'I felt more handicapped from the treatment I received at the hands of hearing people than from my deafness'. Deafness may be a real handicap, but deaf individuals suffer a lot more from our closed minds than they do from their own closed ears.

This is cause for serious concern. Before considering the realities of deaf children's lives, we must first take stock of what prejudices they have suffered in the past and what prejudices they still suffer today.

Prejudice Against Deaf Children

Deaf children who are deprived of articulated speech — simply because they don't hear it — present a paradox to all those around them. For though we may not realize it, we have all been deeply influenced by classical philosophy, which takes thought and word to be intimately linked. Our emphasis on the spoken word as the privileged place of thought goes back to Plato. His system of philosophy defines *logos* as meaning both 'thought' and 'speech', and attributes mysterious power to the latter. Deprived of such vocal speech, deaf children find themselves excluded by society.

In antiquity, the deaf were ostracized, considered cursed by the gods, and stripped of their civil rights. Aristotle barred them from participating in the pursuit of knowledge.

Even in the times of the Abbé de l'Epée in eighteenth century France, deaf children suffered a tragic lot. The following passage comes from a letter written by the Abbé himself:

> Parents looked upon having a deaf-mute child as a disgrace; they believed themselves entirely just toward their child if they provided him with food and shelter; yet they would keep him entirely out of sight, confined to the recesses of a cloister or the obscurity of some unknown boarding-house. (Degérando, 1827: v. I, 10)

Such dramatic prejudice against deaf children was still alive and well in the nineteenth century. In *Camille et Pierre*, published in 1844, Musset tells the story of two deaf-mutes whom people called *demi-vivants* (the half-dead). 'Deprived of speech, they were denied thought', he explains (Musset, 1844: 575).

Today, prejudice based on the absence of vocal speech is not quite so obvious. For instance, we recognize that speech is enveloped by extra-verbal communication and that this extra-verbal communication begins at birth and involves a set of skills specific to verbal communication. But prejudices still exist. They may be less absolute, but they are no less tenacious.

Such prejudices are often the underlying motivation behind professionals' more or less conscious insistence on giving speech instruction *top priority* when dealing with deaf children.

This eagerness to 'make' the deaf speak at any cost can also be explained by a fact we might not want to acknowledge: deafness is a *shared* handicap. Deafness is different in this way from other handicaps such as blindness or paralysis. One doesn't become blind with the blind or paralysed with the paralysed: we can see for the blind to guide them, and walk for the paralysed to transport them, but we can't speak for the deaf.

With a deaf person, we ourselves become 'deaf'; that is, we lose our ability to understand our interlocutor when that person, being deaf, talks to us in the particular manner of someone who cannot hear the sounds of his or her own voice. In describing the situation of a deaf child faced with a hearing interlocutor, Julian de Ajuriaguerra (1972: 237) writes, 'The deaf child is not like a blind person who is seen though he cannot see; the deaf person not only can't hear, but is not heard'. Such a breakdown in the communication process puts both interlocutors — deaf and hearing alike — in the *same* predicament.

In Chapter 1 we showed that all speech is intended primarily for someone other than the speaker and occurs within a relationship of relative positioning and recognition between these interlocutors. Difficulties in understanding a deaf person's speech throw this relationship out of kilter. To make matters worse, a hearing person's speech ceases to come with natural ease to the extent that a deaf interlocutor has trouble deciphering it.

In other words, deaf people are not the only ones put in the awkward and disconcerting position of not being able to guarantee uptake of their speech acts. Hearing people find themselves in the same predicament, for their speech acts may be taken wrongly or not understood at all by the deaf person trying to decipher them. This gives hearing people the sinking feeling that they are out of line and have done something inappropriate — which is hard to take when one is accustomed to easy communication and the sense of the well-being that comes from effortless interaction. This explains why hearing people have trouble approaching deaf children and the handicap of deafness objectively.

Some expressions now used in everyday language betray this lack of objectivity. Take, for example, the French expression *dialogue de sourds* (meaning the kind of 'non-dialogue' that would presumably occur between two deaf people). This expression saddles deaf people with a communication problem that actually arises in dialogue *between deaf and hearing people*. As we will see, dialogue among the deaf themselves is just as effective as dialogue among the hearing.

In sum, prejudice against the deaf stems from the *communication difficulties* that arise between deaf people and hearing people.

Being forced into sharing a handicap does not incline hearing people toward truly accepting the deaf. When they find themselves unwittingly caught in an annoying situation of poor communication, they can't help but want out — and rejecting a situation is just a step away from rejecting the person who brought on the situation.

Deaf individuals are not well accepted in our twentieth-century society — the proof being how little communication really exists between hearing people and deaf people. Just take, for example, professionals who work with deaf children. They object to working alongside deaf adults and shy away from any in-depth interaction with them. They believe that the deaf children they treat will become 'like' hearing people, perfectly 'integrated' into hearing society. Such professionals make a point of keeping the children's hearing parents from meeting any deaf adults at all. In fact, deaf adults are practically hidden from them. The reasoning these professionals use to justify their attitudes goes something like this: 'Parents have it hard enough discovering that their own child is deaf without the added ordeal of meeting deaf adults. Besides, these deaf adults were deaf children in the old days before the latest advances in treatment were made'. As these professionals see it, today's deaf children will become 'just like' other adults, any difference having been erased.

Concerned individuals try to explain that 'what deaf adults want ... is for you to help them become TRUE deaf, not a hybrid with a hearing personality grafted on to a deaf body!' (R.-M. Raynaud, 1978: 2). But their voices go unheard and professionals persist in their denial of deafness.

Consequently, deaf children are raised in a way that negates their handicap and forces them to behave 'like' hearing children. They are accepted and loved only on condition that they behave as though they were not deaf. Such an upbringing completely cuts deaf children off from deaf adults. Some people pretend that deaf adults don't even exist.

But how can we possibly know a child — any child — if we can't imagine who he or she might be in the future? Knowing deaf adults would seem central to getting to know deaf children as they really are. To ignore deaf adults is to ignore deaf children.

But ignoring deaf adults seems to be one way in which hearing people avoid sharing a handicap they find too difficult to bear. Professionals' zeal for 'making' the deaf talk often stems from their desire to deny the handicap and perpetuate their illusion that if they could just make deaf people speak vocally, the deaf would no longer be such disturbing people to talk to. As we have seen, however, a deaf person — cut off from the auditory channel — will never be able speak vocally 'like we do'.

This tendency to obscure the reality of deafness may present certain advantages to the hearing, but it is extremely harmful to the deaf in that it rejects and even negates their very existence. We talk of integrating these individuals while denying them even the right to be deaf. Is it any wonder that the deaf suffer from a real lack of interaction and contact in a society that refuses to acknowledge them as they are?

The vast majority of deaf people are confined to low-level jobs even though they enter this world with the same intellectual potential as hearing people. Just like immigrant minorities — who also fill the lowest-ranking jobs — their real handicap is *cultural*, stemming from their profound isolation from any kind of positive communication with the majority population.

Denying the handicap of deafness results in serious cultural deprivation — a handicap much heavier than deafness itself for a deaf person to bear, but which no longer weighs on hearing people since it does not require their real collaboration.

The child psychoanalyst Eugene Mindel and psychologist McCoy Vernon (1971) (both of whom have a deep understanding of the world of deafness) write in their book about deaf children: 'Most hearing people, however, do not choose to become involved with the deaf because it is often too frustrating' (Mindel & Vernon, 1971: 3). Hearing people refuse to become vulnerable when it comes to what they cherish most in themselves — their ability to communicate.

Behind all of today's humanism and progress in hearing aid technology, what the deaf really live still goes unacknowledged and what they really need isn't 'heard'. How can deaf people experience real interaction with hearing people if they are 'kept at a distance' even when it comes to something that directly concerns them — namely their lack of hearing? Decrying prejudices against the deaf, Hans Furth (1973: 50) explains that 'for too long experts have determined to know what is best for the deaf child and adult without taking into account the real-life situation'.

But there is another way to approach deafness. Instead of fleeing from the handicap, we can acknowledge it and be willing to look at what it implies for our own lives as hearing individuals to engage in true exchange with the deaf and to treat them as real interlocutors.

First of all, it means getting over our initial feeling that communicating with the deaf is 'too frustrating'. Only then can we enter into the world of deafness. This in turn means letting go of our usual ways of communicating and our reassuring yet false preconceptions. As we let go, our feelings of frustration gradually give way to an appreciation for all that the deaf can teach us — both about themselves and about ourselves — through real interaction.

Only once we are willing to 'become' deaf with the deaf and to learn from them can we introduce them to our hearing world; only once we discover the immense richness of their culture can we share the richness of ours.

Taking this approach, we will now focus on deaf children.

Some deaf children are born to parents who are also deaf. We present these children first, for in discovering who they are we also learn something about deaf adults. This view of how deaf children actually live and speak will reveal how utterly unfounded certain notions about deaf children really are.

Deaf Children of Deaf Parents

Fifty to sixty percent of all deafness is hereditary, or the cause is unknown, and ninety percent of all hereditary deafness is carried by a recessive gene. The chances of inheriting deafness are a real 'lottery of genetics';

for 'although this recessive gene for deafness is present in approximately one out of ten persons, only six children per ten thousand are deafened genetically' (Mindel & Vernon, 1971: 25). Genetic probability is such that deaf couples often bear hearing children. In fact, there is only a one-in-four chance that their child will be deaf. 'Most genetic deafness results from the matings of hearing parents' (Brown, Hopkins & Hudgins, 1967: 101). As it turns out, 90% of all deaf children are born in hearing homes. So deaf children of deaf parents are actually the exception.

But this exception offers us a glimpse into how deaf children develop in an environment where their parents are familiar with and acknowledge their handicap. It also affords professionals who know all too little about the lives of the deaf a chance to meet them as they are among their own and at home.

An encounter with deaf parents: the reality of Sign Language

Hans Furth devotes the first chapter of his book *Deafness and Learning* (1973) to a deaf couple and their 'extraordinary ordinary family' because he believes that anyone with a bit of curiosity and tolerance can learn much by observing the day-to-day life of the deaf.

The scene opens with the mother cooking dinner while chatting with an old friend from school. From time to time she checks on her three-year-old-son who is playing in the adjacent room. On one of these occasions her son catches her eye and tells her that he is hungry. His voice is clear and accompanied by a gesture. We take her gestured response, accompanied by somewhat intelligible speech, to mean that he'll have to wait a little while. A moment later the doorbell rings and the child cries out, 'Daddy! Daddy!' pointing to the bell-connected flashing light that lets the mother know when someone is at the door. She opens it to find none other than the father home from work. Happy to be home, he takes his son in his arms and settles down in the kitchen, his son still on his lap, to join in conversation with his wife and her friend. In the course of their discussion about a car accident involving one of their mutual friends, the boy contributes to the conversation now and again.

As they sit down to dinner, everything happens just the way it would in any other home, the only difference being that the happy and animated conversation flows not through mouths but through hands and faces. These individuals are clearly *deaf* but they certainly aren't *mute*. They talk just like ordinary people, in a language that obviously lets them converse like you or I. Meeting these people simply feels like meeting a family who speaks a completely foreign language.

One might be struck, however, by the intensity of their eye contact. These people watch each other with keen attention in order to catch all that is said in their visual language. One might also notice the obvious enjoyment they take in conversing. In each other's company they can finally communicate with ease after a whole day at work in a hearing world where, as the deaf say, more often than not 'eight hours of work equals eight hours of silence'.

'Now that you have glimpsed the life of deaf adults', writes Furth (1973: 5), 'you no longer doubt that deafness is a condition that a person can successfully accept and accommodate to'. He points out that in the United States the deaf are the only group among the handicapped who refuse the tax benefits allotted them. Not wanting any special privileges, the deaf merely ask that they be treated as fairly as anyone else.

Many authors who explore the lives of deaf people come away amazed at their ability to lead productive lives despite their handicap and, more incredibly, despite all the erroneous notions people have about them. These notions are spread primarily by professionals in the field of deafness who remain ignorant of how the deaf really live.

One of the most serious misconceptions about the gestural communication of the deaf consists in refusing to recognize it as a *language*. Up until very recently, future educators of deaf children were still taught that gestural communication is good for only concrete thought and does not help the deaf acquire language. As a matter of fact, Sign Language has been forbidden in schools since the Congress of Milan in 1880!

These misconceptions about signing parallel the misconceptions people have about the deaf themselves. They all boil down to rejection of those who don't hear and who cannot fully participate in vocal communication. How we express ourselves is so much a part of who we are as individuals that *to reject gestural communication is to reject the deaf individuals who use it.*

The fact that the deaf manage to make a life for themselves in the face of such continual rejection has caught the admiration of authors such as Harry Best. He dedicated his book *Deafness and the Deaf in the United States* (1943) to the deaf themselves, calling them 'the most misunderstood of all human children, but the most industrious of all'. By sheer tenacity they have kept their language alive despite the fact that it has gone unrecognized for one hundred years and been forbidden in the schools where they grew up. Sign Language has survived such repression because it is a necessity of life for the deaf. In reality, Sign Language is not what people think it is. In the following section we will show just how unfounded common perceptions of Sign Language really are.

Unfounded preconceptions about Sign Language

Just as classical philosophy linked thought and the vocal word, the science of linguistics emerged in the twentieth century with an emphasis on the vocal nature of language. Listing the criteria that define a language, André Martinet (1964: 29) wrote, 'We must reserve· the term *language* to describe an instrument of communication with this twofold articulation and vocal manifestation'. In other words, no communication among humans by means other than vocal speech could be considered a language.

The fact that the deaf of all countries communicate with gestures had been widely observed. No real studies were conducted, yet this communication was nonetheless declared to be a mere hodgepodge of gesticulations unsuited for the expression of abstract ideas. Linguists maintained that the gestural communication of the deaf was devoid of grammar, and in no way constituted a language. Furthermore, they assumed that unlike the languages of different countries, gestural communication was universal and for the most part iconic, that is, based on images and not on arbitrary signs.

Thus initially discounted, gestural communication was never given any linguistic consideration. The new science of linguistics was to be applied only to vocal languages.

It was only very recently, in the 1960s, that studies by the American linguist William Stokoe led to the discovery that the gestural communication of the deaf fulfills all of the criteria that define a language, other than being vocal. But this last characteristic of language had been established simply through circular reasoning: all languages were assumed vocal because only vocal languages had been studied.

Since Stokoe's ground-breaking work as the father of gestural-communication linguistics, many other linguists have become fascinated with this new field of study that is stretching the horizons of general linguistics itself. They have discovered that *verbal* activity is not necessarily *vocal*. Hearing subjects are comfortable with vocal languages that rely on an audio-phonatory feedback circuit. If we simply open our eyes we can see that the deaf, not having that link, base their verbal interactions on a visual-gestural feedback circuit. They thus enjoy a normally functioning feedback process which, according to Charles Hockett (1958), constitutes one of the fundamental characteristics of all human language.

In his *A Course in General Linguistics*, Ferdinand de Saussure (1986: 7–10) writes, 'The essence of a language, as we shall see, has nothing to do with the phonic nature of the linguistic sign'. Referring to the American linguist

William Whitney, he continues, 'Man, in his view, might well have chosen to use gestures, thus substituting visual images for sound patterns'. Saussure recognizes this theory as perhaps too extreme, for the choice of using the voice organs was not accidental but 'in some measure imposed on us by Nature'. He nonetheless concludes that 'the question of the vocal apparatus is thus a secondary one as far as the problem of language is concerned'.

Thus, even early linguists had some inkling of a fact that wouldn't be established until much later through research on the gestural communication of the deaf, namely that the vocal channel is not the only channel for the word, or speech.

Non-hearing human beings have the genius to realize themselves through speech produced with the hands.

At this point we must redefine a few terms. When general linguistics takes gestural languages into account, the terms *verbal* and *vocal* can no longer be taken as synonymous. *Verbal* refers to speech as a general concept that applies to both *vocal* and *gestural* expression. All speech, be it vocal or gestural, is primarily produced by interlocutors while in each other's presence. But speech can also have a written form for timeless communication outside the space of dialogue — thus the distinction between *oral* language and *written* language. *Oral* is that which is not *written*. When we take into account gestural languages, the terms *oral* and *vocal* can thus no longer be taken as synonymous either. Figure 4.1 illustrates these terminological distinctions.

Many vocal languages do not have a written form. At present, no gestural language has a written form, but it is entirely possible that one could develop.

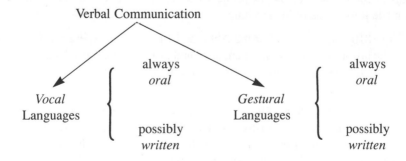

FIGURE 4.1

While the discovery of gestural speech may have been somewhat 'revolutionary' to the field of modern linguistics, it most definitely revolutionized the lives of the deaf. Recognized as having a language, they were at last recognized as complete speaking subjects, and thus as people.

We have seen that no one can 'become' except in and through language. To recognize that the deaf speak a real language — a language no less real for being visual — is to grant them a status identical to that of any other ordinary person and to put them on an equal footing with the hearing. In other words, no longer seeing the deaf as paradoxical subjects who cannot talk, means no longer considering them inferior in their personhood either.

In *De l'éducation des sourds-muets de naissance* (1827), Degérando showed that once the deaf received an education based on recognition of their gestural communication, which was accepted as 'a language of signs, a true, conventional language' (Degérando, 1827: v. I, 18), they were able to enjoy a truly human existence. 'They remained foreigners to us, but they became men' (ibid.: 482).

The Abbé de l'Epée is to be particularly admired because he observed and respected the fact that the deaf communicate with each other through gestures. He even adopted this communication as the basis for his educational methodology. Seeing that the deaf already had a language of their own, he used this language to teach them oral and written French through a process of translation. Accordingly, the Abbé de l'Epée solicited deaf teachers for his school, as did his successor, the Abbé Sicard.

Contrary to common belief, gestural language is not an artificial language at all — the Abbé de l'Epée did not *invent* it. The Abbé was simply an admirable teacher who listened to his deaf pupils, recognized and respected their means of communication as 'the primary path to knowledge', (Cuxac, 1980: 31) and made it the basis of his teaching.

By 1810, 'fifty years after the Abbé de l'Epée's first experience [with the deaf], the history of French Sign Language had grown sufficiently long for interaction among deaf adults to be as rich as among the hearing', asserts Cuxac (1980: 31).

Today, in the 1980s, Sign Language is just beginning to be accepted again after a hundred years of forced obscurity and the deaf feel they are once again becoming recognized as complete human beings. At the first National Symposium on Sign Language Research and Teaching in 1977 in Chicago, hearing linguists shared the floor with many deaf linguists who expressed how much it meant to them that their languages were being studied. Along with other deaf lecturers, Barbara Kannapell — a sociolinguist and president of the Deafpride Movement — explained that once she discovered that her gestural communication had the same status as any other language she finally felt equal to other human beings as a speaking subject. As a deaf child of deaf parents, Kannapell learned very early that she must not use gestures at school even though it was perfectly natural to use them with her parents. She came to believe that signed communication was inferior to English and, by extension, that she herself 'was inferior to a hearing person' (Kannapell, 1974: 11). It wasn't until Kannapell was much older that she discovered, through linguistics, that the gestural communication of the deaf was a true and complete language. This discovery transformed her life. Acknowledging her language meant acknowledging herself and being freed from feeling inferior to hearing people — she too had a language that she could manipulate with ease.

The communication of the deaf has been the object of erroneous and unfounded assumptions that wrongly portray what it really is. Once the deaf are able to divest themselves of these prejudices — which they are made to believe — they regain their identity as speaking subjects, knowing that they stand on an equal footing with the hearing.

The gestural communication of the deaf is not a hodgepodge of gesticulations

In approaching the gestural communication of the deaf linguistically, Stokoe *et al.* (1965) discovered that gestures are organized in the same way as vocal signs in vocal languages — by *double articulation*. Gestural communication, in other words, can be analyzed in terms of *meaningful units* having both a semantic content and a gestural expression; but the gestural expression itself can be analyzed in terms of *distinctive gestural units* unrelated to meaning. Stokoe labeled the meaningful units of the first articulation *kinemes* and the distinctive units of the second *cheremes*. He identified 55 cheremes and found that they could be classified according to three parameters: handshape, placement and movement. Phonologists studying vocal languages similarly classify phonemes in terms of consonants and vowels, adding a third parameter for tonal languages.

According to Stokoe's classification by parameter there are:

(1)   19 cheremes defined by *handshape*. These handshapes correspond, with few exceptions, to those that the deaf use for counting and finger-spelling (each letter of the Manual Alphabet is made with a different handshape). Figure 4.2 shows the French Manual Alphabet along with the handshapes for the numbers 3 and 5. (See Appendices B and C for the American and British manual alphabets.)
       Thus, by referring to a particular letter or number, the handshape of a sign can easily be described. For example, one would say that the sign

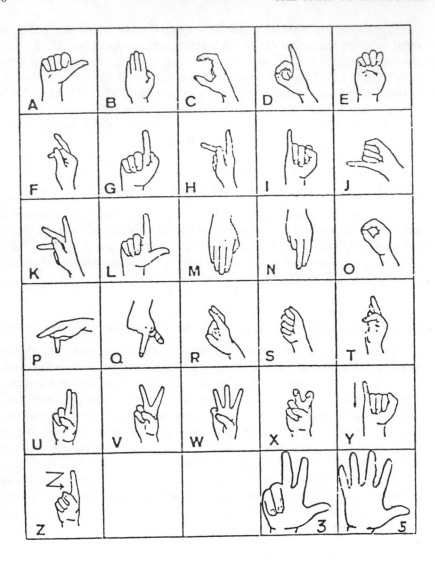

FIGURE 4.2 *The French manual alphabet and other handshapes*

WORK[1] is made with the 'S' handshape, that is, with a closed fist, as in the letter S.

(2)   12 cheremes defined by *body placement* (half-way up the face, at the chin, at neck level, etc.).

(3)   24 cheremes defined by *hand movement* (vertically upward, vertically downward, laterally toward the right, etc.).

As hand movement became better defined, Robbin Battison, Harry Markowicz and James Woodward (1975) found there to be a fourth parameter: *palm orientation*.

Phonological research on American Sign Language thus began with Stokoe's fundamental discovery that signs are doubly articulated. It has since become clear that there are more cheremes than Stokoe's conservative estimation of 55. Before their exact number can be determined, more in-depth phonetic and phonological research must be undertaken. Psycholinguistic research on the psychology of sign formation is also still in its early stages. But given the current state of research in this field, Battison (1978) contends that it is more important to show the validity of Stokoe's parameters than to determine how many cheremes belong in each of them.

In this vein, Ursula Bellugi, Edward Klima and Patricia Siple (1975) conducted a short-term memory experiment comparing hearing and deaf subjects. The hearing subjects were asked to recall lists of words and the deaf subjects (all native users of American Sign Language (ASL)) were asked to recall lists of signs. The results showed that recall errors were not linked to the meaning of the items but to their structure and form. For example the hearing subjects would mis-recall 'vote' as 'boat,' confusing two words that differ only in their respective phonemes [v] and [b]. Similarly, the errors made by the deaf subjects were based on the 'phonological' properties of the signs. For instance they would mis-recall HOME as YESTERDAY. These two signs (in ASL) are identical in placement, movement and orientation, differing only in handshape. Errors also revealed confusion within the other parameters. The fact that differences between the signs recalled and the signs listed were due to a confusion in handshape, placement, movement or orientation validates the usefulness of analyzing signs according to these four parameters. François Grosjean (1979: 56) further contends that these recall errors show 'the psycholinguistic soundness of Stokoe's "phonological" description'.

Recent research by Charlotte Baker (1976) shows that facial expression plays an important syntactical role in American Sign Language and may serve to distinguish lexical units as well. *Facial expression* thus constitutes a fifth parameter.

Every kineme (meaningful unit) thus appears to be defined in terms of *simultaneously articulated* cheremes (distinctive units) belonging to the five parameters mentioned above. As Cuxac (1980: 33) points out, however, 'simultaneity is not unique to sign languages — tones and vowels can also combine at the same point in the chain'.

Researchers studying French Sign Language (LSF) are now finding *minimal pairs* (two signs that differ only in one parameter) that determine which of the five parameters various cheremes belong to. Thus the same parameters seem to provide a very effective means of identifying the basic units of sign formation in French Sign Language, too.

As in vocal languages, secondary articulation units in Sign Language conform to linguistic constraints. The fact that some combinations are not possible makes for specific rules for the formation of signs.

In ASL, for example, Battison (1974) found that two-handed signs are subject to a series of constraints. When both hands move, they must be identical in shape, and either identical or symmetrical in movement and orientation. When only one hand (the dominant hand) moves, the other hand can have one of only six possible handshapes: S, B, 5, G, C, or O (see Figure 4.2). As Battison explains, these particular handshapes are considered the most 'unmarked' and are common to all sign languages studied to date. Interestingly, this law of symmetry and the restriction on hand-shapes also apply to two-handed signs in French Sign Language.

Constraints such as those mentioned above make certain chereme combinations impossible and determine the rules for forming kinemes.

In vocal languages, secondary articulation units interfere with and modify each other by assimilation, dissimilation or metathesis as they are linked together in words and phrases. These same phenomena have been found to exist in sign languages.

In sum, far from being a hodgepodge of gesticulations, sign languages conform to strict rules of formation and share the most basic attribute of all languages: *double articulation*.

As we now focus on units of the first articulation, we will see that they too are organized in specific ways. The notion that sign languages are non-grammatical is completely without substance.

The gestural communication of the deaf is not devoid of grammatical rules

Many believe that gesturing is totally non-grammatical. Yet this idea is based on very superficial examination. Typically, the casual observer looks for a word-for-word correspondence between the sign language and vocal language of a particular country. When there is no such correspondence, the observer concludes that gestural communication must be a mere sequence of movements lacking any kind of internal organization.

Such an approach can hardly qualify as linguistically sound, for 'there is nothing linguistic in the proper sense which may not differ from one language to another' (Martinet, 1964: 20). No one would argue, for instance, that Russian must be non-grammatical because it has a different word order from French and does not have grammatical equivalents for all French words.

Gestural communication has been seriously misconstrued because instead of being considered in its own right, it has been judged on the basis of word-for-word equivalence with vocal languages. Evaluated for what it is not, gesturing has gone unappreciated for what it is.

Because sign languages are based on sight, their structure will necessarily be very different from that of vocal languages, which are based on sound. To properly observe sign languages, we must therefore first learn to open our eyes. Two gestures, for instance, may appear identical (when in fact they are different) because our 'hearing' eyes aren't able to perceive the difference. We must also have an open mind — sign languages use space as their dimension and employ unique space-based constructions, such as *location* and *directionality*, which can be executed simultaneously.

Such constructions make sign languages highly *inflectional*. Lexical units can undergo numerous morphological variations that serve to identify the function of various kinemes. The verb GIVE, for instance, can be signed in a number of different directions to identify the agent and the object of the action. If the sign is made from the signer's body toward the person he or she is talking to, the message is I-GIVE-YOU, but if it is made in the opposite direction, the message becomes YOU-GIVE-ME. To say 'Pierre gives Marie', one would first sign PIERRE in one place and MARIE in another to assign them each a point in space, and then sign GIVE from PIERRE to MARIE. To say 'Marie gives Pierre', one would simply reverse the direction of the movement GIVE between where PIERRE and MARIE are each hypothetically located.

Thus in sign languages, word order is relatively flexible. In saying 'Pierre gives Marie', it doesn't matter whether one signs PIERRE and then MARIE, or MARIE and then PIERRE, because the direction of the verb GIVE is what determines the agent and the object of the action.

Sign Language word order was observed to be different from that of vocal languages long before any linguistic studies on the subject were undertaken. Yet people assumed that Sign Language must be non-grammatical because they were oblivious to the fact that space could fulfill syntactic functions through means of location and directionality.

Incidentally, the vast majority of all signs are made within a defined 'signing space': an imaginary box extending from just above the head to just below the waist, and only so far to either side of the body.

In the example 'Pierre gives Marie', we saw that the direction of the GIVE movement between where the signs PIERRE and MARIE were located identified who was the agent and who was the object of the action. Such identification was possible because PIERRE and MARIE were signed in different places. Now, what happens in a statement such as 'the cat gives the mouse...'? To be signed correctly, CAT and MOUSE must both be placed right near the nose. With both being signed in the same place how can the direction of the verb GIVE be established? The signer resorts to a process called *indexing*: upon signing CAT and MOUSE, he assigns each a respective point in space. Those two points then serve as pronouns between which the GIVE movement can be performed.

Sign languages use indexing extensively. Once a sign has been made and assigned a location, one can refer to it for the remainder of the conversation by simply indicating its assigned spot. Points in space thus serve an anaphoric function. They are usually referred to by pointing, but the signer can also designate them by a look of the eye. This type of spacial locating is basic to a number of grammatical structures now being studied that will further reveal how space is used for syntactic purposes.

As we have seen, the verb GIVE can take on many different directional variations that serve to identify possible agents and objects. At the same time, it can also undergo another series of morphological variations that indicate various aspects of the action. Sign languages are very rich in expressing this type of nuance. For example, Carlene Pederson (1979), a deaf linguist at the Salk Institute, made an inventory of all the ways TO BE SICK could be signed in ASL. She identified a morphological variation for each of the following nuances in aspect: SICK FOR A LONG TIME, JUST FELL SICK, OCCASIONALLY SICK, OFTEN SICK, SLIGHTLY SICK, VERY SICK, CHRONICALLY SICK. Such inflections follow regular forms and constitute a variation paradigm that can be applied to many different kinemes that function as verbs.

Research shows that French Sign Language expresses aspect in the same way. Cuxac (1980) has identified ten different inflections applicable to all verbal kinemes:

> Some, such as the imperfect and the progressive, are frequently found in oral languages. Others are more rare, such as the repetitive and the 'staccato'. And some can only be paraphrased as 'secretly', 'slow progressive', 'promptly', 'affectedly', etc. Since a perceptive verb such as SEE can incorporate some fifty different inflections of this type, we will classify those forms that don't apply to other verbs as derivations (Cuxac, 1980: 36).

Such pioneering syntactic research shows that if we examine sign languages in their own right — not in terms of what they seem to lack compared to vocal languages — we find that they are organized according to a complex grammar. This established, we can now attack a third misconception, namely that gestural communication is essentially pictorial or iconic.

The gestural communication of the deaf is not universally understood 'transparent'[2] *pantomime*

At first glance, the most striking feature of the gestural communication developed by the deaf is the imagery of signs. For instance, once a person is told how to say 'cat' in French Sign Language, the sign seems obvious, for it clearly suggests a cat's whiskers: the hands start in an 'O' handshape (see Figure 4.2) at either corner of the mouth, then open up to extended fingers as they move horizontally outward to ear level. By contrast, the corresponding linguistic sign in spoken French, 'chat' [ʃa], does not evoke any relationship to the animal at all.

Similar observations have inspired such labels for the gestural communication of the deaf as the French *le langage mimique* (miming language) or *le langage mimo-gestuelle* (gestural miming language). Such labels suggest that this kind of communication is more akin to transparent pantomime than to a language. Yet the facts belie this view. For instance, a hearing person observing two deaf people talk to each other in gestures cannot understand their conversation.

Notice also that these labels use the French term *langage* rather than *langue*. The first term, *langage*, means 'language' in a general sense whereas the second term, *langue*, means a specific language and describes 'the different modalities of language as a universal human phenomenon' (Martinet, 1964: 18). These labels serve to perpetuate the notion that the gestural communication of the deaf is universal.

Research by Klima and Bellugi (1979) on the iconicity of signs used in American Sign Language shows that the meaning of ASL signs can rarely be guessed, whereas that of pantomime is always obvious. Ten hearing people with no knowledge of American Sign Language were presented with 90 signs by deaf native users of ASL and asked to guess what they meant. For 81 out of the 90 signs, no correct answer was given by any of the subjects. The notion that signs are 'transparent' is thus completely without substance.

In another experiment, the subjects were asked to choose the correct meaning of signs by multiple choice among four possible answers. This obviously made the meaning of the signs much easier to grasp. Yet still only 12 of the 90 signs were correctly answered by a majority of the subjects.

By contrast, when the subjects were given a list of signs with their meanings and asked what *relationship* they saw between each sign and its meaning, they gave identical answers for over half of the signs and tended to see the same kind of connections. For instance, they all saw the sign WOOD as a sawing motion that seemed to link the sign with its meaning. Our example of someone learning how 'cat' is said in French Sign Language reflects this same phenomenon.

Although signs are not 'transparent', we could say that they have a 'translucent' quality to them that links certain characteristics of their form with their meaning. 'Certain aspects of ASL signs can recall certain aspects of their meaning. But their pictorial nature is never so unambiguous that someone who doesn't speak ASL could guess their meaning (even when the correct meaning is provided among several possibilities)' (Klima & Bellugi, 1976: 527). We must also keep in mind that while the form of certain signs might suggest their meaning when listed in isolation, they usually lose this quality when they occur in the flow of speech and interact with other signs. When produced in isolation, the sign HOUSE, for example, does suggest the shape of a house. But when it occurs within the flow of speech, it looks more like an open bridge. Furthermore, sign languages are highly inflectional. This means that regular morphological variations can be applied to any sign and completely obscure its translucency within an utterance.

Finally, we must also recall that signs are made up of regular units upon which all sign formation is based. For example, the sign CHAT is formed with a particular *handshape*, *placement*, *movement*, and *orientation*, each of which is a unique unit of secondary articulation in French Sign Language. This secondary articulation ensures the arbitrariness of signs. With respect to spoken languages, Martinet (1968: 28) asserts that 'phonemes, the product of the second linguistic articulation, are what guarantee the arbitrariness of the sign'. The fact that gestural signs are arbitrary, however, does not impinge on their pictorial or iconic qualities. This iconicity may completely disappear in the flow of speech under the arbitrary rules of sign formation and the morphological variations of grammar, yet it nonetheless remains a typical characteristic of sign languages. In fact the deaf take advantage of this feature in various discourse situations. They purposely bring out the imagery of signs in poetry, for instance, which is a form of discourse that plays on the materiality of the linguistic sign. The iconicity of sign languages is also more pronounced in the special speech register used to address young children just learning to speak gesturally.

In Chapter 1 we argued that speaking is both *saying* and *showing*: semantic signs serve to represent and to show. Sign languages — visual languages *par excellence* — best demonstrate the semantic sign's dual nature as both a *sign* that represents and an *opaque thing* that shows itself.

The iconicity and arbitrariness of the semantic sign are not contradictory. Sign languages play heavily on iconicity, yet they remain arbitrary languages that vary from country to country and which cannot be understood by those who do not know them. They certainly can't be reduced to some transparent, universal pantomime. In referring to the gestural communication of the deaf, we thus prefer the term *langues des signes* (sign languages) over *langage gestuel* or *langage mimo-gestuel* because these last two expressions suggest a universality that doesn't exist and are based on a false perception of sign language as meaning-transparent pantomime.

Although sign languages differ from one another just as vocal languages do, they might also show similarities when their histories have been intertwined. Such is the case for the French and American Sign Languages. In 1816 a deaf professor from the *Institut Royal des Sourds de Paris*, Laurent Clerc, travelled to the United States to help Thomas Gallaudet open the first American school for the deaf. He brought with him his teaching methods — based on those of the Abbé de l'Epée — and French Sign Language, which was flourishing at that time. The language of course underwent rapid transformation within the American deaf community, yet to this day there remain great similarities between American and French Sign Language. As justice would have it, the French now benefit from the relative proximity of the two languages (150 years after Clerc made his contributions in the United States). Today, the many linguistic studies conducted in the United States on American Sign Language generally apply to French Sign Language as well.

In this section we have shown that preconceived notions about the visual-gestural communication of the deaf are unfounded. We have also shown that the gestures of the deaf actually constitute languages that are no less real for being visual. Now we will define the role that these languages play in the personal development of the subjects who speak them — namely, the deaf.

Sign languages are the only languages that allow deaf people to enjoy all of the characteristics of speech

We have established that sign languages are indeed true languages. Now we will show that they are the *only* languages that let deaf people develop positively as complete speaking subjects. Because they are based on vision, sign languages offer deaf people unhindered, handicap-free verbal communication as no other language can.

As pointed out in Chapter 1, no 'statement' can be interpreted outside of its enunciation and the fact that it is said: the *connecting process* between the interlocutors is basic to any interpretation of the 'statement' (the content of what is said). Only sign languages let deaf people enter into this fundamental connecting process without obstacle. The connection is achieved visually, in a language that permits a *normal process of linguistic communication* — a language that lets deaf individuals take their place as full-fledged speaking subjects just as hearing people do in vocal languages.

In Chapter 1 we presented all that speech is from the perspective of the speaking subject. The following review of each of those characteristics clearly shows that only sign languages can offer deaf people speech in all its fullness.

Speaking is hearing, expressing and identifying oneself

All speech is produced under constant monitoring by the utterer through a process of internal feedback. For a hearing person who speaks vocally, this feedback is provided by the sense of sound — speaking is hearing oneself.

Through Sign Language, a deaf person can also experience the internal feedback of his or her speech, which is based on a visual-gestural circuit. Feedback is provided by the sense of sight — speaking is seeing oneself.

Sign languages are the only languages that offer deaf people linguistic communication with complete internal feedback. When using a vocal language, a profoundly deaf person receives only partial feedback — sometimes hardly any at all. Speaking vocally is a real feat for a deaf person, but not one that necessarily fulfills all of the characteristics of linguistic communication.

Speaking is also expressing oneself. Again, a deaf person can experience this aspect of speech only in a language based on visual feedback. When speaking in a visual-gestural modality, deaf people can express themselves verbally without the least difficulty or handicap. Unhindered by any sensory limitations, they can modulate and play with their speech just as hearing speakers do by playing with sounds.

Another feature of linguistic communication that we have discussed and that holds true for deaf people only in sign languages is the fact that the physical nature of signs produced and signs received is identical. That is, regardless of whether one is sending or receiving a message, the nature of the linguistic signs conveying this thought remains the same. In vocal languages these signs are auditory in nature — Saussure (1986: 98) calls them 'sound patterns', and in visual languages they are visual in nature and result in 'visual patterns'.

When deaf people use vocal language, they produce signs based on kinesthetic sensations (for lack of auditory feedback) and receive signs based on sight (since words can't be heard they must be 'read' on the speaker's lips and face). In other words, when the deaf 'speak' in a vocal language they are truly performing a great feat, for the nature of the signs they produce and receive are not identical. Thus their 'speech', for all it is worth, does not match the characteristics of linguistic communication.

Only in interactions in Sign Language is it possible for deaf people to produce and receive signs of a consistent nature and experience the richness of speech as a means of identifying with others.

Speaking is also finding one's place

We have seen that speaking is also receiving and assuming a place within the interpersonal relationship of a spoken interaction. In relating her own experiences (see page 32), Armengaud explains that as a deaf person she finds it impossible to assume her place in a vocal conversation, particularly when it involves more than two people. There is no way she can fully participate in a conversation designed to be heard — not 'read' (i.e. visually deciphered). In fact she usually gets only the 'skeleton' of the conversation. Under certain conditions a deaf person might, with enormous effort, manage to follow a conversation and want to join in, but often it's too late and the comment seems out of place.

Only sign languages offer deaf people visually-based conversations in which they can fully participate. With all barriers to the interpersonal connecting process removed, they can then find their place in the conversation; that is, they can assume their place as a speaking subject, and from that place speak up and be recognized. That act of recognition is what enables a deaf person to 'say something', for no statement can be made outside of an exchange relationship in which each of the interlocutors is recognized.

Without a gap between the 'fact of saying' and 'what is said', deaf people demonstrate a perfect command of all the conversational rules of discourse. In the nineteenth century, at a time when Sign Language was flourishing, the deaf organized banquets with debates and speeches and proved to be very gifted orators. During this period in France, deaf poets and writers produced works in French. Since they knew where they stood in Sign Language, they were able to command a greater place in the society and language of the hearing than deaf people do today. Because of their visual speech, they knew that they were full speaking subjects.

Speaking is becoming a subject

Research on language development in deaf children of deaf parents has shown that these children go through the same stages learning to speak (in a visual mode) that hearing children go through. In fact Marina McIntire (1974) and Ronnie Wilber and Michael Jones (1974) have found that deaf children of deaf parents generally utter their first words (in sign) two to three months earlier than hearing children do (McIntire, 1974; Wilber & Jones, 1974). These authors attribute this earlier emergence of language in deaf children of deaf parents to the fact that hand muscles mature faster than tongue muscles do. Like ordinary children, these deaf children quickly advance to two-word utterances. McIntire (1974) observed one deaf child who had a twenty-sign vocabulary and made two-sign utterances at just ten months old. At that age, most ordinary children are just getting ready to say their first word.

Since sign languages are the only languages that let deaf people experience speech in all its fullness, they are also the only languages that enable them to *develop normally* and without delay as speaking subjects.

A deaf person who has been kept from Sign Language is someone who has never even experienced true linguistic communication. Such individuals blame themselves for their vocal communication difficulties and believe that they simply don't have what it takes to speak. Little do they realize what an exploit it is that they communicate vocally at all! Since they have never had access to true linguistic communication in a language in which they are not handicapped, they also have no way of knowing that their vocal speech accomplishments — despite the enormous skill they require — will never be the means to reaching their full verbal potential or to satisfying their communication needs.

Deaf people who simply cope with vocal language, experience unending frustration as human speaking subjects. And this constant state of frustration interferes with their self-image. The repeated failure they experience attempting to communicate vocally makes them feel like a failure themselves and think of themselves as inferior. Besides being hampered in their speech, they become hampered in their personal development.

This observation illustrates, albeit in negative terms, the fact that humans come to exist in and through speech. Depriving deaf people of Sign Language (the only language that lets them really speak) amounts to seriously debilitating them as whole individuals.

Forbidding the use of Sign Language cannot be compared to prohibitions against minority languages, such as the Breton or Basque languages in France. Prohibiting Breton may be detrimental, but those deprived of this language can nonetheless acquire another vocal language and thereby fully develop their linguistic abilities. This is not true of deaf people deprived of Sign Language.

Deaf people who haven't been kept from Sign Language know what it means to communicate linguistically. They understand what causes their difficulty with vocal language and know that the problem does not lie with them as speaking subjects. In other words they can distinguish their own linguistic abilities (which are intact) from the difficulty of carrying on a verbal exchange in a vocal language that they cannot hear. Simply put, they understand the true nature of their handicap and the fact that deafness hampers them in vocal languages but not in visual languages. These deaf people know that they are full speaking subjects and that they possess a language in which they can 'become' without any obstacles in the way — just like hearing people. As far as language goes, feelings of inferiority are unknown to them.

Only through Sign Language can deaf people gain a clear sense of their identity both as *deaf individuals* and as *complete speaking beings*, for this is the only language that lets them develop as healthy speaking subjects.

It shouldn't come as any surprise that, as Moores' (1978) research has shown, deaf children of deaf parents (who are exposed to Sign Language right from the crib) grow up with a real advantage over deaf children of hearing parents. And what is the situation of deaf children born into a hearing family? This is the question we will now consider.

Deaf Children of Hearing Parents

During their first year of life, deaf children of hearing parents enjoy multisensory communication with their mother just as all children do when all goes well.

But this multisensory communication does not revolve around vocal language. Deaf children do not hear the vocally spoken words that accompany all that their mother communicates to them through her eyes, face, gestures, etc. A mother's vocal utterances are so 'situation specific' that even without hearing them, deaf children can still fully participate in these first exchanges. They respond to their mother and sometimes even initiate interaction through their own eyes, expressions, gestures, and babbling (which continues for the first three months).

Sight plays such an important role in mother-infant interaction during the first year of life that all children grasp and understand messages more through what they see than through what they hear. All the while, however, the ears of hearing children are soaking up linguistic information based on the sense of sound. Deaf children do not experience this aural and verbal saturation which is so essential to acquiring vocal speech.

Somewhere between six and twelve months a mother usually begins to sense that something is missing in her multisensory interaction with her baby.

Her baby actively engages in dialogue based on movement, motor games, smiles, etc., but shows no interest in voice games. As Eugene Mindel and McCay Vernon (1971: 42) write: 'Contrary to general opinion, most parents of a deaf child develop a definite conviction that their child is deaf by the time he is six months of age. Often, this is not articulated. But the sense that the child does not hear is there'.

Despite her strong suspicion that her child is deaf, the mother still hopes that her fears will prove unfounded. She thus goes through a very painful period once the deafness is actually diagnosed.

As we saw in Elizabeth Wilson's case (see page 76), once a mother receives the audiological test results, she tends to see her child no longer as an *infant*, but as *deaf*. In studying parental reactions to the diagnosis of their child's deafness, the psychosociologist Katheryn Meadow (1966) found that hearing parents are more distraught over their child's inability to *speak* than over the child's inability to *hear*. Because mothers perceive their deaf child as being incapable of talking, they themselves become incapable of talking to their child. As seen earlier, maternal speech is a response and an adaptation to child speech. If the child doesn't speak, the mother feels at a loss, deprived of her ability to communicate. A breakdown occurs in the mother-infant communication that was developing normally in a multisensory mode as long as the mother had no idea that her child was deaf.

The shared handicap of communication

When deafness is diagnosed in a child, it is the mother who 'loses' her speech. The knowledge that her child is deaf squelches her anticipation of the infant's speech and makes her feel that she can no longer connect with her baby — her words won't get through. Consequently, she herself becomes communicationally handicapped, unable to speak naturally to her child.

As long as a mother remains unaware of her child's deafness she can dialogue and communicate with her infant perfectly well. She understands what her baby is telling her in his or her own special way, and she knows that her baby understands her. Between them there exists true interaction based on multiple senses. But because she overestimates the importance of vocal speech to this exchange, the discovery of deafness leaves her completely undone.

When this happens deaf children must suddenly deal with much more than their own deafness and the deprivation of verbal communication that it has imposed since birth: they must also face their mother's distress. With that distress comes a break in their normal way of communicating and a near total loss of the *extra-verbal communication* that used to envelop their mother's 'statements'. 'I can't look at my child without despairing', one mother confessed as she experienced the pain of no longer knowing how to communicate with her child.

What kind of support is there for mothers who are distressed because their child doesn't speak?

The diagnosis of deafness sweeps parents (especially mothers, who are generally more available) into a medical and paramedical world that focuses exclusively on *hearing loss* and the resulting *absence of speech*. This explains why children are fitted with a hearing aid as soon as their deafness is diagnosed.

All a hearing aid can do for a profoundly deaf child is make audible a few noises or sounds, usually in the low frequency range. This is practically of no help at all when it comes to the fine-tuned and nuanced acoustical qualities of speech transmitted in the 500 to 4,000 hertz frequency range.

In short, profoundly deaf children cannot pick up the sounds of speech through a hearing aid. In the best of cases, the hearing aid helps them become aware of their own voice. They may continue to babble, thereby maintaining a quality of voice that might later make it possible for them to speak vocally with proper pitch. This is by no means insignificant. But it does not allow for spontaneous acquisition of vocal speech. The subtle acoustical qualities of speech still go unperceived.

Consequently, deaf children usually start receiving speech training at the time that they are fitted with a hearing aid. Such 'early intervention' is aimed at encouraging them to make sounds and focus their attention on the sensory stimulation of speech: the visual stimulation of 'lipreading', the tactile stimulation of body vibrations, and whatever auditory stimulation the hearing aid provides. Mothers are shown how to talk to their young child in a way that provides such stimulation. They are informed, for instance, that they must talk right in front of their child so that he or she can see their facial movements.

In sum, everything possible is done to enable deaf children to communicate vocally and to get them to speak.

The support that parents receive — mothers in particular — all centers on attempting to remedy their child's vocal language deficiency. It would seem, then, that mothers' expectations are met, for what distresses mothers is the fact that their deaf child doesn't speak. They believe that communication will 'get back to normal' once their child can speak and re-become for them a speaking subject.

But it does not work out that way, of course. The hearing aid and 'early intervention' might succeed in teaching their deaf child to speechread a few words and even produce some, but that hardly makes for normal family communication. What seemed an appropriate response to the family's distress simply doesn't work. When the parents show consternation at their child's slow progress and the problems they have communicating with him or her, they are advised to be patient and persevering — after all, it takes a lot of long, hard work to 'get' a deaf child to speak.

So parents live out the first years of their deaf child's life in a spirit of despair as they wait and hope for the normal speech and communication that obviously won't be forthcoming since the child cannot hear.

It is not uncommon, notes R. Thomas (1979: 11), to find '6 and 7-year-old deaf children who have the vocabulary of a 15-month-old hearing child (25 to 50 words) and not nearly the language comprehension. *They cannot communicate*, and suffering such terrible frustration, they throw fits of anger, have bouts of depression and exhibit behavioral problems'. At the age of seven, one young profoundly deaf boy could only speak one word: [meʒ], meaning *méchant* or 'mean' — an insult he used on his mother every morning when she came in to wake him. This was his way of expressing his rage and frustration at the non-communication he was still enduring despite his nearly life-long speech training. How could his mother communicate the tenderness and confusion she felt? Facial expressions and lipreading could not go very far in helping her and her child overcome their shared handicap of communication.

What support mothers and their deaf children receive through vocal speech training simply isn't enough. While intentions of teaching a deaf child to speak vocally may be laudable and even useful, they can be dangerous if they become the sole focus, with nothing else done to reestablish satisfying mother-child communication.

As shown earlier, ordinary children begin to learn to speak in an atmosphere of communication: mothers seek first and foremost to establish dialogue based on what their child does. If in interacting with her deaf baby a mother mainly emphasizes vocal speech, the whole language acquisition process breaks down because the mother is insisting on something that her child can neither spontaneously produce nor even easily perceive. Stressing vocal speech actually keeps deaf children from being able to communicate. Yet communication is the very foundation and starting point of linguistic interaction. And furthermore, it is not through vocal speech that a deaf person can ever experience linguistic communication in all its fullness.

In sum, mother-infant interaction focused exclusively on vocal speech actually handicaps deaf children linguistically, as well as communicationally, for their linguistic abilities cannot fully blossom in a vocal modality.

It often takes parents two to three years of 'early intervention' before they realize that although their child (now three to five years old) can 'say' a few words, still no linguistic communication has developed between them. It's the deaf child and the child's family who pay the price for this realization: they are the ones who live the non-communication and suffer from it more deeply with each passing day.

Effects of the communication handicap on the psychological development of deaf children

If made to grow up in an atmosphere where everything focuses on correcting for something they lack, namely the ability to speak vocally, deaf children suffer enormously. The few vocal words they do manage to produce and recognize with years of hard work hardly satisfy their communication needs.

Jurgen Ruesh (1957) has shown that healthy psychical development cannot occur in children who suffer communication problems. A mother who doesn't understand or know how to respond to what her child is trying to convey causes that child confusion, frustration and anxiety.

If the child is deaf, the mother is likely to feel frustrated, too. She tries her best to grasp and respond to what her child is telling her — practicing that amazing maternal pedagogy discussed earlier. Yet for all her desire she still fails to understand her child or, if she does understand, fails to respond in a way that her child can understand. As a result, the mother gets frustrated trying to communicate with her child. Furthermore, it pains her to be causing her baby such suffering by being unable to understand or make herself understood. Imagine how hard it must be for a mother to *have no words* with which to calm and comfort her baby in situations that are difficult and incomprehensible to a child — such as a separation or moving to a new home.

By seriously dampening the atmosphere of mother-infant interaction, such communication difficulties end up affecting children's psychical development. Frustrations, tensions and misunderstandings inevitably come out sooner or later in the form of behavioral disorders.

Children who have suffered in this way are prone to extreme fits of anger and to withdrawal symptoms not unlike those associated with various psychoses. In fact a large percentage of profoundly deaf children have been labeled 'psychotic' at some point in their life. Such children also tend either to rebel or recoil when adults try to reach out to them.

Professionals encourage parents to treat their deaf child as they would any other, communicating essentially through vocal speech. But the fact is, deaf children who are spoken to vocally do not grow up to be like children who can hear vocal speech.

A study by Katheryn Meadow, Hilde Schlesinger and Constance Holstein (1972) compares the behavior of 40 deaf children aged thirty months to four years to that of 20 hearing children of the same ages. All the deaf children were of hearing parents and all had a hearing loss of over 80 decibels in the conversation range (500–1,000–2,000 hertz). None presented any other handicap. The children were videotaped for 20 minutes each in interaction with their mother. Each mother-child pair was invited to play as they wished with blocks, trucks and dolls, and then asked to engage in more structured activities such as looking at a set of picture cards, drawing on a blackboard and sharing some refreshments.

The deaf children appeared to be much less happy than the hearing children during interaction with their mother. Deriving less pleasure from the interaction, they were also less creative and less capable than the hearing children. These observations also showed that mothers of deaf children behave very differently from mothers of hearing children, tending to be less flexible than other mothers in interacting with their children. In fact the mothers of deaf children displayed very controlling, authoritarian and didactic behavior — behavior 'designed or intended to teach'. Thus, for instance, instead of enjoying playing with their child, they seized upon free play with the blocks as an opportunity to have their child practice the names of colors.

The authors of this study partially attribute the behavior of these mothers of deaf children to the advice they receive from experts on deafness who focus exclusively on vocal speech. The point is to talk: if you talk to your child your child will talk back. Every situation thus becomes an opportunity to 'teach' speech, often without any room for the pleasure and purpose-free indulgence so essential to communication and language development. Every aspect of the mother-child relationship ends up crystallizing around the vocal speech the child is lacking — the very thing the child is least capable of because he or she doesn't hear.

The above study also revealed another interesting fact: contrary to what one might suppose, mothers of deaf children do not communicate gesturally with their child much more than do mothers of hearing children. Again, this probably reflects advice received: always try to use vocal speech to communicate with your child.

No wonder deaf children appear to be less happy than hearing children when interacting with their mothers. Besides having a hard time communicating, they can never live up to their mother's expectations. All their mother seems to care about is vocal communication — something utterly beyond the grasp of a little child who can't hear.

The disappointment that deaf children see in their mother's eyes hardly makes for a positive self-image or sense of worth. Hearing children, on the other hand, know that they are 'big' and 'smart' in their mother's eyes. They know they are her pride and joy.

So in addition to putting a damper on the interaction and communication that speech requires (thereby disturbing the language acquisition process), the emphasis on vocal language deficiency also disturbs the whole mother–child relationship.

Authors such as Eugene Mindel and McCay Vernon (1971) explain this fixation on vocal speech as an attempt to make young deaf children blend in: 'Talking' makes them 'normal', no different from others. But this is to deny deafness and deny the child's handicap. As we saw at the beginning of this chapter, hearing people hide behind their denial in order to avoid sharing a handicap that would affect their usual way of communicating.

In Moores' view, the advice that parents receive is dangerous: it centers exclusively on vocal speech and is offered by

> well-meaning but misinformed individuals[3] whose advice has not really been aimed at the healthy development of the deaf child but rather at the neurotic selfish needs of parents who want their children, as psychological and physical extensions of themselves, to be 'normal', that is, speaking. (Moores, 1978: 98)

In sum, parents get caught up in making the rounds of medical and paramedical services that do nothing to help them receive their child as a unique and different individual. 'That fixation on normalcy (speaking) prevents parents from working through their grief to the mature acceptance of deafness that is a prerequisite to adequate psychological and social development' (Moores, 1978: 98). Deaf children are thus put through unnecessary suffering. How can any child bloom and be happy if not accepted for who he or she is?

Such obvious suffering and injustice snaps some parents out of the abnormal situation into which they and their child have been plunged. In the following account, one set of parents explains that their three-year-old deaf daughter's ever-deepening sadness and withdrawal finally made them speak up and question what was happening.

> With difficulty she could say a few words — 'bread', 'drink', 'goodbye'. But no new words came in their wake. The speech therapist's long-promised

breakthrough was nowhere in sight. Aurélia was over 3 years old and *still no system of language had developed between her and us — her parents...* We were led to believe that it would be easy to communicate through various different means: drawing, mime, lip-reading, articulating, and all the rest. Were we so communicationally insensitive that we couldn't succeed in these things that seemed so simple? Was establishing a relationship with a deaf child as easy as those nice people in speech therapy made it out to be? (Maigre-Touchet & Maigre-Touchet, 1979b: 259)

These parents, recognizing the lure they had fallen for, looked at their daughter and said, 'We had foolishly hoped that you would talk as we do, you who are profoundly deaf, you who can't hear and can't make out but a few low sounds' (Maigre-Touchet & Maigre-Touchet, 1979a: 13).

Through a painful process — all the more painful for the false hopes they had entertained — these parents finally embraced their little girl and her handicap and asked themselves what might be 'normal' for her. They began to notice what was special about their daughter. They also became a real family. The child gained an identity — she was deaf — and her parents regained their role as parents which, above all, is to communicate with their child. By truly acknowledging their young daughter's handicap, they discovered how to communicate with her in a modality that was not purely vocal.

Other parents, too, have been through the process of acceptance. Thomas Spradley (1978) tells of his experience:

> *Normal.* That word had haunted us from the moment we learned of Lynn's deafness. 'You want your child to be normal, don't you?' It had driven us to talk, talk, talk. Now we began to ask a different question.
>
> 'What is normal?' From Lynn's perspective, nothing had been normal. Least of all the kind of communication skills we had expected her to learn. *A deaf child's idea of normal cannot possibly coincide with a hearing parent's idea of normal.*
>
> By denying her deafness and treating her as if she were normal, we actually made her feel different. Even in the most ordinary family activities, by talking as if she could hear when she could not, we created for her the profound feeling that she was on the outside, a stranger to what was going on. Only after we began to sign regularly did we realize how the pretense of normality had appeared to Lynn. For the first time in her life[4] she did not merely sit at the table watching our mysterious lips, seeing us laugh and smile for unknown reasons. She began to share the day's activities. (Spradley & Spradley, 1978: 249)

Spradley's account shows that the enormous mental suffering deaf children of hearing parents experience is due not directly to their deafness but to being treated 'as if they could hear'. Such treatment stems directly from the advice of professionals who do not concern themselves with the realities of deaf children's lives.

Before we can teach deaf children, we must know who 'deaf' children really are. 'Deaf' means 'does not hear'; it does not mean 'does not speak'. We must not look at nonhearing children exclusively in terms of their vocal speech deficiency but in terms of what they really live. Children are children whether they hear or not. They all have the same needs and the same ability to communicate and speak. Only once we truly acknowledge this identity in deaf children can we offer them the same chances of blossoming that we offer other children.

Conclusion: Deaf Children Are Complete Speaking Beings

The fact that deaf children cannot spontaneously acquire vocal speech does not mean that they cannot speak.

As we have seen, deaf children of deaf parents acquire language in the same way that hearing children of hearing parents do. The language they speak is a *visual* one that lets them develop as speaking subjects and communicate without any handicap at all. Within their deaf family they lead a perfectly normal life.

But professionals who deal with deafness completely disregard this fact; they simply deny that there is any such thing as a deaf person who is different in ways that can never be erased when it comes to vocal communication. They refuse to acknowledge the existence of a deaf population, and even avoid the term 'deaf': the children they treat are *hearing impaired* or *hard of hearing* — not at all similar to those 'gesticulating' deaf adults who weren't fortunate enough to benefit from new hearing aid technology and speech rehabilitation techniques.

Professionals have been encouraging this separation between deaf children and deaf adults for decades now. The deaf adults whom professionals today dismiss as 'yesterday's deaf' are the same children who passed through their very hands not so long ago.

Just like other hearing people, professionals try to negate deafness completely, fleeing from a reality they find too unsettling because it might require that they reexamine their own way of communicating and speaking.

As a result, parents do not receive any support toward accepting their child's handicap. Instead, they are led along a course of education that in the long run turns out to be disastrous in that it completely negates their deaf child, whose difference and true identity go unacknowledged.

Opening a two-day seminar on 'The Deaf: From Childhood to Adulthood' in June 1978, R. -M. Raynaud, president of France's national confederation of the deaf, addressed the assembled professionals saying,

> ...I would ask you to remember that in approaching the deaf and the problems inherent to their condition, one must try to get beyond his or her own preconceptions. Whenever this has been done, a spectacular increase in results has been obtained, particularly qualitatively. Simply put, never ignore the handicap by trying to make the deaf into hearing people. (Raynaud, 1978: 2)

Our approach to deaf children is aimed at 'getting beyond our own preconceptions' by listening to the deaf themselves. They alone can help us to understand better what it means not to hear. The most important realization we must come to is that *not hearing* and *not speaking* are in no way connected: the deaf have a visual language in which they are able to reach their full stature as speaking subjects.

Hearing parents experience great relief when they find this out. 'Deaf' no longer has to mean 'mute' — quite to the contrary. At long last they are free to embrace their child's handicap and difference, for they no longer perceive their child only in terms of vocal speech deficiency. In fact they discover that, in a visual mode, their child can express him or herself beautifully.

Parents can then *identify* with their child, no longer seeing him or her as being strange — a mute, incapable of understanding and being understood. They know that in a visual language their child is capable of expressing him or herself and communicating without the least handicap, just as they do.

This recognition allows children to get past their auditory handicap and once again become their parents' pride and joy; and it allows parents to become parents again, enjoying healthy communication with their child.

Even though deaf children are full speaking subjects, they cannot access language unless they go through the same necessary processes other children do in appropriating speech. Like all children, deaf children need a privileged person — usually their mother — with whom to acquire language through satisfying communication and easy, enjoyable interaction.

Deaf children, too, have the right to a mother tongue. But how can they be given one? This is the topic of Chapter 5.

Notes to Chapter 4

1.   All words printed in small capitals refer to their corresponding kineme, i.e. a word in Sign Language.
2.   Here we use the term 'transparent' to mean iconic. This is not to be confused with Récanati's use of the term as discussed in Chapter 1.
3   What makes this so serious is that these people are professionals in the field of deafness.
4   Lynn was five at the time.

5 Deaf Children's Access to Speech and their Right to a Mother Tongue

We cannot determine what leads to healthy speech development in deaf children until we have defined who 'deaf children' really are.

In Chapter 4 we defined deaf children to be complete speaking beings with the same language and communication needs as other children. The challenge, then, is to create for them a learning environment that offers the same essential conditions of speech acquisition that other children enjoy.

To review, we learned in Part One that ordinary children start acquiring speech right at birth through the very special preverbal and verbal interaction they have with their mother.

Simply by following their instinctive 'pedagogy', mothers are able to *anticipate* their infant's communicative abilities and *communicate* with their infant in preverbal dialogue and verbal conversation. It is through such multisensory mother–infant interaction that the *mother tongue* emerges and the infant gradually begins to communicate verbally. But what about deaf children? How can they be given access to speech?

In our presentation of deaf children we pointed out that 'deaf' does not mean 'mute'. This means that a mother *can* anticipate her deaf child's ability to communicate. And her anticipation is crucial, for it restores the fundamental basis of language acquisition in children. Knowing that her child is able to communicate and express him or herself without any handicap at all in a visual language, the mother no longer feels hindered in her 'anticipatory illusions' about her infant's communicative abilities. She comes to understand that her child, while handicapped hearing-wise, is not handicapped in communicating visually. In fact, the child's communicative abilities are fully intact. Realizing this, the mother no longer sees her deaf infant as a child who *doesn't speak* but as one who simply *doesn't hear*.

This realization creates a much more conducive atmosphere for speech acquisition in that the mother recognizes her child as a full partner. She understands that her deaf infant is a speaking being who urgently needs to begin *communicating verbally*.

But this process will differ depending on whether the child's mother does or doesn't hear. Deaf children from hearing families, in other words, will have a different *mother tongue* from that of deaf children from deaf families. For this reason, we will consider each situation separately.

The Mother Tongue of Deaf Children of Deaf Parents

Deaf children of deaf parents are born into a family that knows about deafness from personal experience. In such a home, a deaf child is nothing new.

Not all deaf parents know that their gestural communication is a true and complete language. But those who do know feel fulfilled as parents in that they have a language they can pass on to their children. It may be a minority language, but it nonetheless provides easy and relaxed communication within the family (barring any extenuating material or social or psychological problems at home). Such parents want their children — deaf or hearing — to learn both their own visual language and the majority vocal language. They want their children to fit into both of the worlds in which they live: the world of the deaf and the world of the hearing.

As we know, babies begin to acquire speech right at birth. Accordingly, we will observe how deaf mothers interact with their infant during the first months of life (before they might know for sure whether their child is deaf or hearing).

We are able to study deaf mothers' first interactions with their deaf babies thanks to research conducted by Julia Maestas y Moores (1979). Maestas y Moores recorded 40 videotapes ranging from ten minutes to one and a half hours in length. The vast majority constitute a longitudinal study of four infants from the age of 0 to 6 months interacting with their parents during play, feedings and baths. Three other infants were also videotaped in similar settings, one at 11 months and the other two at 16 months. Given the age of the infants, most of the recordings are of mother–infant interactions, but a few interactions involving fathers were also videotaped.

When Maestas y Moores presented a number of these recordings at the Copenhagen Seminar in August 1979,[1] researchers observed that, like hearing mothers, these deaf parents were doing everything they could to create fun and relaxed *communication* between themselves and their infant.

Like hearing mothers, deaf mothers converse verbally with their infants as they draw them in to preverbal dialogue. They also take advantage of all the senses — touch, sight and sound included — to establish communication with their baby. In almost no time at all, the infant begins to initiate preverbal dialogues as well. In sum, deaf mothers employ the very same strategies that hearing mothers do as described in Chapter 2.

During such interactions though preverbal communication, deaf mothers bathe their babies in visual speech — and also in vocal speech. For instance, Maestas y Moores (1980: 7) observed one deaf mother sign MILK several times in a row to her baby, and in between each repetition also vocalize the word 'milk'.

In verbal exchanges with their infants, deaf mothers have also been observed to speak in a particular manner paralleling the variations of the special child-directed speech register (see page 54). First of all, their speech matches the discursive strategies unique to this register. Everything they say to their child is clear and closely linked to the context in which it is uttered. As for syntax, deaf mothers produce well-formed sentences while not avoiding certain complex structures. And phonologically, they adapt their speech the same way hearing mothers do, that is, they speak in a slower rhythm so that their child can clearly distinguish what they are saying.

Some phonological variations used by deaf mothers are unique to Sign Language. First, they tend to make signs right on their infant's body to help him or her internalize their placement through tactile stimulation. For instance Maestas y Moores recorded one mother signing CUTE on the chin of her 25-day-old son rather than on her own, as the sign would normally be made. Deaf parents use this technique all the time. 'Signing on the body of the infant is a strategy common to all the parents', asserts Maestas y Moores (1980: 5). Secondly, deaf mothers often model their infant's hand or hands into the correct handshape of a sign and guide them through the proper movements. One mother was videotaped doing this to help her five-month-old son sign DOG, MOMMY, and DADDY.

Deaf mothers also talk to their infant in the same kind of 'free-flowing speech' that we described in Chapter 2. At times they don't care whether or not they are understood, but simply ramble on in their child's presence as though he or she were an extension of themselves. In sum, deaf mothers offer their infant the same kind of *language immersion* that hearing mothers do. Using visual language, deaf mothers talk to their baby both in a special speech register and in free-flowing speech.

As a result, children of deaf parents enjoy trying to produce signs themselves just as children of hearing parents enjoy trying to vocalize words. In one interaction videotaped by Maestas y Moores we see a deaf mother sign 'Are you full?' to her 25-day-old son, Arturo, after nursing him. After attentively watching his mother sign FULL, Arturo makes a rough attempt to reproduce the sign.

Children of deaf parents also play with signs in the same way that children of hearing parents play with sounds. In fact deaf parents tell their children nursery rhymes and lullabies in Sign Language. They know how physically pleasing signifiers can be in a gestural language and how much children enjoy the poetry of harmoniously flowing signs.

A videotape of a little deaf girl named Donna at 16 months and 3 days shows the kind of linguistic communication that had developed between her and her father even at this young age. About a year older than the other children whom Maestas y Moores videotaped, Donna takes a much more active role in initiating communication and produces many signs that are perfectly understandable even though she doesn't sign them exactly as an adult normally would — just as hearing children learning to speak deform vocal words, so deaf children deform signs. For example, she doesn't use the normal hand shape for the signs CAT, FROG, AIRPLANE, PLAY or SHOE in American Sign Language. In signing CAT, she extends all of her fingers instead of dropping the index to meet the thumb in the proper 'F' handshape (see chart in Appendix B). Yet her sign is understandable because she makes it with the correct placement and movement (Maestas y Moores, 1979).

This same videotape shows Donna using the techniques that adults use when they address young children. At one point she signs YOU on her father's body, and at another takes his hand and moves it through the sign DOG.

At 16 months, most children can't yet make two-word statements, yet here we see Donna produce sentences containing several signs:

THROW ME THAT
BOOK DOG BOOK
MOMMY NO SHOE
PLAY TOGETHER
DOG WHERE?
THAT, WHO? MOMMY THAT

Like hearing children, deaf children's first words are quickly followed by two and three-word statements. And very early, they begin to use little interrogatives. 'It is very interesting that in this videotape Donna uses the questions "where?" and "who?" at only 16 months' (Maestas y Moores, 1979: 96).

In short, this deaf girl of deaf parents was able to acquire language at a very young age because, right from the crib, she enjoyed a *mother tongue* that drew her into a visual language in which she was completely free of any handicap at all.

In Chapter 3 we discussed Halliday's observation that mothers 'track their child's language'. Studies have shown that this is also true of deaf mothers. From a very young age, they interpret certain of their infant's hand and mouth movements as the child's way of 'saying' something. 'Mothers read semantic intent into the infant's hand configurations, actions and/or locations at a very early age', explains Maestas y Moores (1980: 10), citing the example of one mother who saw in her two-month-old baby's way of moving and placing his hands the signs AIRPLANE and SLEEP. Maestas y Moores (1980: 9) also observed a mother inferring the word 'milk' from her infant's lip movements without voice at three months of age and 'hello' at five months.

Such observations clearly show that deaf mothers seek to 'understand' their child before they attempt to make themselves understood, offering their own way of expressing something in Sign Language and sometimes also in voiced words, as documented in some of the videotapes referred to above.

Children of deaf parents thus receive their *mother tongue* in a healthy atmosphere of multisensory communication just as hearing children of hearing parents do. To paraphrase Halliday (1979): Before the mother's signs come the child's gestures. By responding to these gestures, deaf mothers give their infant the satisfaction of being *understood*.

Figure 5.1 illustrates this *mother tongue*, that is, the exchange of 'languages' that occurs between a deaf mother and her child (who expresses him or herself in his or her own way).

While deaf mothers adopt the same, truly remarkable linguistic 'pedagogy' that hearing mothers do, they show even greater resourcefulness in their linguistic approach, offering their child not one but two verbal models. They naturally

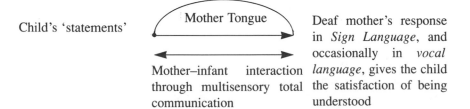

Child's 'statements' — Mother Tongue → Deaf mother's response in *Sign Language*, and occasionally in *vocal language*, gives the child the satisfaction of being understood

Mother–infant interaction through multisensory total communication

FIGURE 5.1

put greater emphasis on their visual language, yet they still give their young child the rudiments of vocal language so as to convey the importance of the lips and voice. Incidentally, this behavior in deaf mothers attests to the 'normalcy' of deaf people's linguistic abilities.

Deaf mothers offer their infant a *mother tongue* that paves the way to two different languages: *Sign Language* (used within the family) and *vocal language* (used in the larger environment). Figure 5.2 illustrates how this *mother tongue* opens up the closed dual relationship between a deaf mother and her infant.

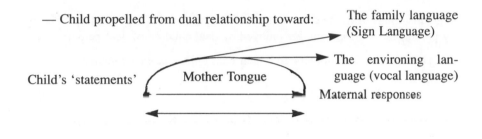

FIGURE 5.2

Whether deaf or hearing, children of deaf parents are nurtured to become *bilingual*.

If deaf parents have a hearing child, they take care to expose that child to hearing relatives and friends on a regular basis or else enroll him or her in a child-care program. This allows the child to develop vocal language alongside the Sign Language used at home. Since hearing children of deaf parents don't experience any handicap in either language, many become bilingual very quickly, and intuitively speak one or the other language depending on whether they find themselves in a deaf or hearing environment. In fact the vast majority of Sign Language interpreters are hearing children of deaf parents.

If, on the other hand, deaf parents have a deaf child, they take care to provide that child with vocal speech training as early as possible, for they know how useful vocal speech can be when it comes to participating in the world of the hearing.

Right from birth, deaf children of deaf parents have a certain advantage: their parents know who they are and what they need in terms of language and communication. (They, too, were once deaf children.) Far from being deprived of communication, deaf children of deaf parents are exposed to two languages in their infancy. The first is Sign Language, which they acquire at the same age that other children (who have enjoyed healthy communication) begin to speak. In fact, as we have seen, deaf children of deaf parents sometimes pick up language even a bit earlier than ordinary children do. Secondly, deaf parents encourage their deaf children to learn vocal language. As Meadow's (1966) study comparing 56 deaf children of deaf parents with 56 deaf children of hearing parents shows, those of deaf parents actually succeed in learning vocal language better than do those of hearing parents. It is only natural that deaf children who begin learning a language at birth and enjoy healthy family communication should have an advantage over those who have not.

This brings us to the critical question of how to offer deaf children of hearing parents the same advantages enjoyed by deaf children of deaf parents.

How can hearing mothers give their deaf child a *mother tongue*?

The Mother Tongue of Deaf Children of Hearing Parents

Deaf children born into a hearing family are born into a family that knows nothing about deafness, and with this ignorance comes a host of preconceived notions about deaf people and Sign Language. Deaf children and their hearing families suffer infinitely more from society's ignorance about deafness (particularly that of the professionals advising them) than they do from the actual deafness and its true consequences.

But things don't have be this way!

If, at the time that their child's deafness is diagnosed, parents are told about deafness and the realities of their deaf child's life, the child can remain for them just that — a *child*, a complete speaking subject. As we showed in Chapter 4 they won't perceive their child (who simply doesn't hear) as someone who *does not speak* and will learn to only with a lot of time and trouble. In other words, they will not perceive their child only in terms of the *vocal* speech he or she is lacking. Instead of thinking of their child as nothing more than a blocked ear — as depicted in the 'Life in Families with Deaf Members' poster for the 1978 World Congress in Copenhagen — they embrace their child as a whole person.

Once parents understand deafness, they no longer experience their deaf child as an incomplete or undeveloped being but as a unique child who, because of the unique life experience that deafness imparts, will develop unique abilities, such as talking with one's hands.

Upon learning that their deaf child has a marvelous ability to communicate visually and lacks nothing in the way of communicative abilities, parents recover their own ability to communicate with their child. Their deaf child once again becomes for them a child whose communicative abilities they can anticipate. As shown earlier, children need this *attitude of anticipation* in their parents before they can begin acquiring language — and deaf children are no exception.

When hearing parents find out that deaf children of deaf parents enjoy comfortable and easy communication with their family through a *visual* language that deaf children can learn without delay, they want this same kind of communication for themselves and their own child. They no longer accept the painful situation in which communication is impeded simply because it is based exclusively on *vocal* language that their child cannot hear.

Discovering the visual language of the deaf gives hearing parents new hope for communicating with their own deaf child — their child may have troubles speaking vocally, but nothing prevents them as parents from learning to speak visually.

In their desire to better communicate with their young deaf child, hearing parents start seeking out *deaf adults* willing to teach them their language. And upon meeting deaf adults they suddenly discover a whole new world — a world they find reassuring rather than frightening.

Here, in their own words, is the experience of one set of parents:

> A few dedicated speech therapists arranged for us to have dinner with some deaf people — deaf adults, that is. We avidly picked up from them what signs we could — they were so expressive and beautifully concise! And meeting some deaf adults helped us to imagine what Aurélia would be like when she grew up. We realized that she would have the same difficulties speaking that they did. If meeting deaf adults convinced us of one thing, it was that oral language by itself was inadequate.
>
> The more deaf adults we met and the more our vocabulary of signs grew, the more we became convinced of something else as well: the deaf are just as much a part of society as anyone else. They have their own language just like Bretons or American Indians and all other people who, because of their local dialect, are bilingual. What a revelation! Now there was no looking back. We knew we had to give Aurélia (who is profoundly deaf) Sign Language. This was *her* language, the language of the deaf — the people with whom she would associate for the rest of her life. We, too, would learn this language and finally be able to communicate with her. (Maigre-Touchet & Maigre-Touchet, 1979b: 260)

In an open letter to Aurélia these same parents write: 'We didn't know how to have a meaningful relationship with you, but now we've really become your parents. And you must feel that signs gave you a mother and a father.' (Maigre-Touchet & Maigre-Touchet, 1979a: 14)

Through Sign Language, this mother and father were able to again become real parents to their deaf daughter and to better understand who she really was. Here is how they describe the impact of their first Sign Language class:

Hands danced against the light; fingers began to move and describe things and meet each other; hands and fingers were talking to us. And you know what? We understood them! In those two intense hours we learned to tell each other our names and other things about ourselves. But more than that, we finally understood the absence of sound. (Maigre-Touchet and Maigre-Touchet, 1979b: 261)

Besides helping hearing parents to imagine their child later on in life (which is vital since children's very essence is in their 'becoming'), meeting deaf adults also helps them to realize that visual language is what frees deaf people to really express themselves and fully exist.

As we saw in Chapter 4, getting to know deaf people means getting to know their language; and getting to know the language of the deaf leads to a better understanding of deaf people themselves — the two cannot be separated. Once parents realize this, they can then offer their deaf child a positive upbringing in a healthy atmosphere of communication.

But this brings us back to our crucial question: How can hearing parents go about giving their deaf child a *mother tongue*?

First of all, they must realize that vocal language isn't going to let them start communicating with their child right away. They need to begin learning Sign Language from deaf adults.

As a visual language, Sign Language uses grammatical procedures entirely different from vocal language; it thus has a completely different structure. Like other languages, Sign Language takes time; it cannot be learned overnight. For hearing people, learning a visual language can be even more difficult than learning a vocal language: more attuned to sound than sight, their eyes don't know what to look for.

Yet hearing parents can gain enormous insights even from their very first Sign Language class. They experience the 'absence of sound' for themselves and begin to realize how much can be said with hands, eyes, the face and the body *without* using the voice. In short, they become aware of *extra-verbal communication* and of the fact that being deprived of vocal words does not necessarily mean being deprived of communication altogether.

Deaf Sign Language teachers take care not to use their voice or refer to vocal language at all when they teach. The point is to initiate their hearing students to *visual communication* and help them become aware of the visual phenomena they normally overlook because they are caught up in the way vocal exchanges *sound*. In the process of showing their students the importance of eye contact and helping them to develop their visual attention, deaf teachers familiarize their students with various features of Sign Language.

Gil Eastman, Dean of the Theater Arts Department at Gallaudet University, has found that the first sessions of beginning Sign Language classes are based more on extra-verbal communication than on communication in Sign Language. Deaf teachers like Eastman try to impart to their hearing students the 'special and remarkable' communication abilities (Moody, 1979: 223) that deaf people display in conversing with deaf foreigners whose language they do not know. In such situations each interlocutor leaves behind his or her own language in order to achieve mutual understanding on the common ground of expressive gesturing — for which the deaf have an incredible knack.

Right from their first class sessions, hearing parents of deaf children find great comfort in realizing how important extra-verbal communication really is. Once they *experience for themselves* what their child perceives in the eye gaze, gestures, faces and so on that envelop vocal words, their attitudes undergo a complete transformation. They then understand the ways in which their deaf child is able to understand them and make him or herself understood. The atmosphere of visual communication experienced in class thus restores parents' ability to talk to their child.

In these renewed beginnings of dialogue, as mother and child enjoy their first conversations with each other, the child enters into the *mother tongue* process. If the child's parents continue in their Sign Language classes, they quickly acquire a working vocabulary of signs. They may be far from fluent in the language, but at least they can accompany their vocal words with signs when they talk to their child.

This small step leads to a qualitative leap in parents' communication with their child. They find themselves marveling at their young child's appetite for language and his or her ability to communicate. As Aurélia's parents write:

Aurélia was learning as fast as we were. We were so exited to be able to tell her the names for things. Our first great rush of emotion came when we realized that Aurélia didn't even know her own name. She immediately latched on to the name-sign that we had 'discovered' for her. Realizing that she had a name, she knew that others must too. That's how daddy, mommy, grandma, grandpa, 'Aïda' [her sister], and others 'came to exist' for her.

We were stunned by Aurélia's memory. She would come out with signs that she had learned days before after seeing them only once. What a change this was from trying endlessly to drill our words into her! (Maigre-Touchet & Maigre-Touchet, 1979b: 261)

Signing allows deaf children to acquire language naturally in an atmosphere of linguistic communication. It reestablishes for them a *mother tongue* — the experience of a real exchange between their own language and their mother's (as they express themselves in their own way, their mother responds, speaking both vocally and in sign). Since their mother's response is conveyed visually as well as vocally, they are able to take it in and make it their own.

Deaf children of hearing parents thus experience the *mother tongue* as shown in Figure 5.3.

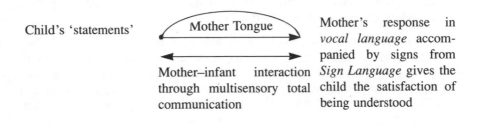

Child's 'statements'　　　Mother Tongue　　　Mother's response in *vocal language* accompanied by signs from Mother–infant interaction *Sign Language* gives the through multisensory total child the satisfaction of communication being understood

FIGURE 5.3

In sum, hearing mothers can offer their deaf child a *mother tongue* and experience the joy of their child's 'first words' just like mothers of ordinary children. They, too, can know the 'miracle of communication' that Perron-Borelli (1976: 690) experienced when her hearing daughter spoke her first word, 'yne-yne' — that one word in which both mother and daughter knew the satisfaction of having unmistakably and unequivocally communicated as never before.

When Aurélia's parents began to learn Sign Language she was already three and a half years old and was linguistically ready to soak up all she could get: '...she acquired and reproduced signs after seeing them only once', marvel her parents (Maigre-Touchet & Maigre-Touchet, 1979b: 259). She also had a 'voracious appetite' for names — she had hungered for them for years!

Another mother tells of a similar experience. She discovered that her son was deaf when he was but three months old, but the doctors didn't confirm this until he was 20 months. She then began using signs when she talked to her infant. He 'soaked them up like a sponge', she exclaims (Thomas, 1978: 8). Even at just 20 months this baby (not having vocal words) was hungering for ways to communicate. In no time at all he had picked up all the signs his mother could offer him and by the time he was two and a half he communicated like any healthy toddler:

> J. says in signs the same precious things that a hearing two-year-old says in words. He tells me when he is angry or sad, and when he feels sick or has hurt himself. He asks me to explain things and we read stories together... He expresses himself in signs with his brother and sister, his father, the neighbors. He is a member of the family...a 'normal' child. Now that he understands what a language is, he has started trying to articulate words, too. (Thomas, 1979: 12)

Deaf children can acquire language without delay provided that their parents do everything possible to ensure healthy family communication through sign-accompanied vocal speech. On 5th March 1980 at the University of Paris, Dr Hilde Schlesinger, Director of the University of California Center on Deafness in San Francisco, presented videotapes of deaf children who had received a *mother tongue* from their hearing parents right from the crib. We might take as an example the profoundly deaf little girl named Jennifer who was regularly videotaped with her mother from the time she was five months old until she was three.

At five months we see Jennifer's mother talk to her daughter in the same kind of multisensory exchange that any mother might have with her child, the only difference being that she accompanies some of her words with signs from Sign Language.

At ten months Jennifer has blossomed and is very attentive to gestures and faces. Her mother shows her a book and explains it to her by speaking vocally and using signs. We see Jennifer roughly sign the words MILK and DOG, and observe her mother exclaiming how happy she is that her daughter is beginning to communicate in a visual language.

At 14 months Jennifer knows 35 signs and is able to combine two signs, saying for example, 'WHERE, TREE?' We might recall that Donna, a deaf child of deaf parents, was observed using WHERE? and WHO? in a similar way at 16 months (see page 12).

By 17 months Jennifer knows 107 signs. Her mother tells us how good their communication is, comparing Jennifer to her other children, who are hearing. She even has the impression that Jennifer is better at expressing her feelings and desires than the other children were at her age. Jennifer's mother says how happy she is that she and the rest of the family took the trouble to learn Sign Language (which is 'so beautiful') so that they could communicate with Jennifer by signing as they spoke vocally.

In her 1979 article 'Deafness and Mental Health' (based on her observation of these same videotapes while on sabbatical assisting Dr Schlesinger), psycho-analyst Françoise Berge substantiates the fact that a deaf person's 'mental well-being' is closely linked to his or her ability to communicate effectively.

When we talk to children who don't yet know how to speak, we address them in a *special speech register* to make our vocal utterances as clear as possi-ble (see Chapter 2, pp. 52–64). Adding signs to one's vocal utterances when talking to a child who doesn't hear arises from this same concern for making oneself understood.

Parents who use signs as they speak are following the same *natural process* that all parents use to talk to a child who doesn't yet speak. That is, they take full advantage of all their deaf child's senses in order to convey a verbal message. By using signs as they speak, they offer their deaf child a *mother tongue* through which he or she can acquire language.

As we have seen, the *mother tongue* (an exchange of 'languages' between the child's self-expression and the mother's response in the language used by herself and others) plants the seed of separation that allows children to move beyond the dual mother–infant relationship. In the case of deaf children of hear-ing parents, this separation comes in the form of several languages.

The first of these languages is the mother's way of communicating with her child by signing as she speaks vocally. This modality, called *Signed French*, is also used by the rest of the family to communicate with the deaf child and to talk with each other when he or she is present — deaf children need to be able to pick up family talk going on around them. Just like all children, they acquire language by being immersed in words — those spoken around them as well as those spoken directly to them.

When hearing parents see how thirsty their child is for communication and language they realize that, like themselves, their deaf child needs to meet deaf adults and needs the language they speak — *Sign Language*. Learning this lan-guage may be a long process for the parents as hearing adults, but their deaf child, being so young, will be able to acquire it very quickly.

In fact, Sign Language is the one language that deaf children can imme-diately acquire without any handicap at all — and meeting deaf adults gives them the chance to do so. But in order to acquire any language they need to have experienced a *mother tongue*. This is true of all children. In Chapter 3 we saw that many hearing children don't ever feel accepted in their own way of expressing themselves — don't experience a *mother tongue*. And this is why they don't learn to speak.

Sign Language meets deaf children's linguistic needs better than Signed French can. Even though Signed French involves signs, it is still essentially a vocal language meant to be heard. Moreover, Signed French doesn't always come easily to parents. Without a doubt, Signed French does improve parent–child communication magnificently. But it does not enable deaf children to communicate with their hearing parents as comfortably and easily as if they themselves could hear.

Deaf children experience such unhindered linguistic communication only when conversing in Sign Language with other deaf people. They must not be deprived of such communication, for it alone can offer them all of the characteristics of speech as described in Chapter 4 on page 103 and following.

To acquire Sign Language, deaf children need to have an on-going relationship with one or several deaf people. These relationships also help them to develop a sense of identity and understand what makes them different — both essential steps toward blossoming as an individual. Aurélia's parents wanted their daughter to meet deaf adults just as they had, and that is how she came know who she was: '...you realized that you were deaf like Nasser[2]; you also realized that daddy, mommy and Aïda were hearing' (Maigre-Touchet & Maigre-Touchet, 1979a: 14). Through these contacts Aurélia became aware of the fact that the world is made up of people who hear (like her parents) and people who do not hear (like Nasser and other deaf people she met). She continued to identify with her parents just as all children do, but she also began to identify with people who were deaf like herself.

By identifying both with their hearing parents and deaf adults, deaf children come to understand that they may speak in signs with deaf people, but must speak vocally with hearing people whom they see talking without signs, only with lip movements — which is what vocal words seem like to them. This is how deaf children begin acquiring their third language — standard *French*.

Hearing parents naturally want their deaf child to be able speak vocally (and they have every right to). They are thus delighted to discover that, by growing up in such home, their child develops the desire to learn to speak vocally without gestures despite the difficulty it presents. It is by speaking vocally that deaf children identify with their parents and other hearing people around them.

To summarize, once hearing mothers understand the nature of their deaf child's handicap, they realize that their child can reach his or her full potential as a speaking subject if offered speech in a visual mode. Having recovered their 'anticipatory illusions' about their child's speech, they regain their own ability to speak with their child. They talk to their child, accompanying their vocal words with visual signs, and thereby reestablish mother–infant interaction based on

verbal as well as extra-verbal communication. Figure 5.4 shows how the resulting *mother tongue* propels the deaf child of hearing parents from the purely dual
mother–infant relationship into several languages.

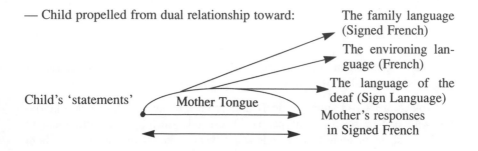

FIGURE 5.4

Through their *mother tongue*, deaf children begin to communication with
their family in *Signed French* (a mixture of two languages — French and French
Sign Language). This modality serves as a *communication bridge* between deaf
children and their immediate hearing entourage. A hearing family with one or
several deaf children becomes a world where deaf and hearing live together
under the same roof. In such a world, Signed French can meet everyone's needs
and include every family member in a shared process of communication. It also
allows the parents to become parents again in that they are able to offer their
deaf child the most normal communication possible.

Such healthy family communication prepares deaf children to acquire *Sign
Language* and *vocal language*. Once they do, they have at their disposal three
different modes of speaking corresponding to the three different exchange situations in which they might find themselves: exchanges with other deaf people,
exchanges with hearing people who know Signed French, and exchanges with
hearing people who speak only vocally. This third exchange situation is of
course the one that deaf children access last of all.

In sum, for a mother to offer her deaf child healthy communication she
must first recognize that Sign Language is the one language in which her deaf
child experiences no handicap. As one mother put it: 'To reject signs would have
been to reject my deaf child'.

At an even deeper level, a mother must first accept what makes her child different — that her child doesn't hear — before she can possibly give that child a *mother tongue* and the chance to acquire the various speech modalities that he or she will need in life.

Far from being speechless subjects, deaf children are destined to know several languages. In conclusion to this chapter, we will further explore why this is so.

Conclusion: Deaf Children Are Destined to Become Bilingual and Bicultural

All deaf children, whether of deaf or hearing parents, are bound to move between two worlds, namely, the world of the hearing and the world of the deaf.

Deaf children of deaf parents are born into a home where Sign Language is spoken. But outside the home they come into contact with another language, a vocal language. Their parents want them to learn this second language as well, for they know from experience that it is the key to hearing culture and to becoming part of society in general.

Deaf children of hearing parents, on the other hand, are born into a home where people speak vocally. But once hearing parents understand that muteness is not a corollary of deafness and once they realize that their deaf child, though hindered in vocal speech by the obstacle of not being able to hear it, *can* acquire a visual language, they want their child to have this language and want to be able communicate with him or her through it. This necessarily leads them to invite deaf people into their lives (not just theirs but their child's as well). As a result, deaf children of hearing parents encounter the same two worlds that deaf children of deaf parents do, and their hearing family serves as a bridge between the two.

As part of acknowledging what makes their child different, hearing parents give their child the right to a different kind of speech — the speech that the deaf use among themselves.

All deaf children are thus destined to become bilingual and bicultural. They become *bicultural* in that they belong to two different communities — deaf and hearing — each of which has its own culture, that is, its own way of seeing things and its own values to live by. While not making value judgments about either culture, we must nonetheless recognize their existence as two distinct sociological realities. One of the most striking cultural differences between the two communities is their respective modes of linguistic communication. For deaf children being bicultural means being *bilingual*. They must be able to wield different languages depending on the situation they find themselves in.

Here we should define exactly what we mean by 'bilingualism', for this word has taken on very different meanings at different times. At the turn of the century bilingualism was defined as equal mastery of two languages. Today the term is used much more generally to denote, 'the alternate use of two or more languages' (Mackey, 1976: 9). Thus defined by William Mackey, bilingualism is nothing unusual, for 'there are thirty times more languages than there are countries to harbor them' (ibid.: 14). These figures (which incidently do not account for sign languages) reveal how intertwined bilingualism and language itself have been down through the ages. It is quite doubtful that any linguistic group has ever existed that did not undergo some kind of exchange with other linguistic groups. Rather than being the exception, bilingualism has always been the norm.

Bilingualism is also often a function of one's level of education. In many countries 'being educated means being bilingual' (Mackey, 1976: 18). Also, some kinds of knowledge are acquired in specific languages — sometimes just knowing how to read the language is sufficient. A person who knows a second language, if only in its written form, is still considered bilingual. According to Mackey's definition of bilingualism, the vast majority of the world population is thus bilingual, for most people know two or more languages.

In this light, deaf people who speak their visual language with ease and are able to read the written form of a vocal language are indeed bilingual even though they may experience difficulty with vocal interactions, since these occur in an auditory modality.

Recognized for who they are, deaf children are destined to become bilingual individuals who use one or another language (vocal language or Sign Language) according to the various linguistic contexts they are sure to encounter.

To consciously and consistently encourage such bilingualism in deaf children, however, we must provide them with a language-learning environment in which each of their two languages is clearly acknowledged *as a language*. Kannapell, who grew up with both American Sign Language and English, believed that her gestural communication was not a true language. She never realized that she had two languages until she went to college and learned in her classes that the gestural communication of the deaf is in fact a true language. Knowing this, she was finally able to accept herself as a deaf person and feel she had a place in hearing society. This point cannot be overemphasized. Only through consistent and intentional bilingualism are deaf individuals able to gain a sense of their own identity and participate in the respective cultures of the two worlds to which they belong.

Researchers have determined that growing up in a natural bilingual environment does not cause ordinary children any language problems. Julian de Ajuriaguerra (1974: 342) maintains that 'from the angle of thought organization, knowing that an object is equal to itself even though it is called by different names can only reinforce the reality of the thing'. When bilingualism is lived out in a natural way (i. e. when each language is used consistently according to context and when they are both equally valued within the family) it cannot possibly harm an ordinary child — quite to the contrary.

While true bilingualism is linguistically harmless for ordinary children, it is linguistically necessary for deaf children. Only through bilingualism can deaf children acquire speech naturally, for it exposes them to a visual language in which they do not experience any limitations in the language acquisition process.

As far as deaf children are concerned, bilingualism is the only road to healthy speech development.

We must emphasize once again, however, that for deaf children to experience real bilingualism, Sign Language must be recognized as a true language. Having a respect for this language is what allows parents to embrace their deaf child as unique, and offer him or her a *mother tongue*. From there, deaf children can go on to become bilingual subjects, learning to communicate linguistically in Sign Language on the one hand and in vocal language on the other.

In Parts One and Two we have laid the theoretical foundation for a new approach to deaf children and deaf education. We now know that the only way deaf children can blossom is through *bilingual education*. In Part Three we will present our pilot program in which we put this theory into practice.

Notes to Chapter 5

1. A NATO-sponsored Sign Language Research Seminar (August 21–29, 1979) that brought together researchers from 16 different countries.
2. Nasser was a deaf adult who visited the family regularly to teach them Sign Language.

Part Three:
A Pilot Classroom: Toward Bilingual Education for Deaf Children

Our examination of speech and how ordinary children acquire it (Chapters 1–3), and our comparison of this with speech and speech acquisition in deaf children (Chapters 4 and 5) all clearly point to the need for a new approach to deaf education.

Parents must be helped to understand the nature of their child's handicap as soon as deafness is diagnosed. They need to know that deaf children can speak and communicate even though they cannot hear — provided that Sign Language is accepted as a true language. Familiarity with Sign Language allows parents to establish satisfying communication with their deaf child while also orienting him or her toward two languages: that of the deaf community and that of the hearing.

This is precisely the approach advocated in 'An Open Letter to Parents of Deaf Children' (Bouvet, 1979a), which appeared in numerous specialized publications including those put out by associations of the deaf and associations of parents with deaf children. As the letter was circulated, something new began to happen: deaf people began regularly visiting hearing families and tutoring parents in communication with their deaf child. Such contacts continued to multiply, enabling more and more parents to reestablish healthy family communication by becoming familiar with the basics of a language accessible to their child — i. e. the language of the deaf. These visits had the added advantage of helping hearing parents understand their child's needs and experiences better, and thus of helping them embrace their child as different. By interacting with deaf adults, hearing parents came to accept their child's handicap. They saw how similar deaf people's lives were to their own and realized that deafness didn't necessarily keep a person from leading a normal life. Meanwhile, the deaf children in these families quickly gained a new sense of well-being as communication was restored and they were given the opportunity to identify with deaf adults. Commenting on such deaf/hearing contact, Bernard Mottez and Harry Markowicz (1979: 68) write: 'It gives young deaf children a deaf role model and helps reassure anxiety-ridden parents that deaf adults are normal people'.

Those families lucky enough to have a deaf tutor found the experience very encouraging. Yet such arrangements were not recognized by the medical and paramedical services that track deaf children and their families. These professionals were generally resistant to the idea of collaborating with deaf adults or of acknowledging their language.

Consequently, only those parents who happened to hear about deaf tutors were able to take advantage of such opportunities. Some managed to find out through newspaper clippings, by word of mouth from other parents, or from one of those rare professionals open to this approach. But to actually avail themselves of a tutor, parents had to surmount more than just an information barrier; they had to stand firm in the face of conflicting advice from the myriad of specialized institutions that provide education for deaf children. Even though much of this advice was unsound — a reflection of how superficial professionals' approach to deafness can be — it still caused parents to agonize over their decision. Thus, even when parents heard about opportunities to meet with a deaf tutor, it wasn't always easy for them to take this step. In addition, families had to pay for the tutor themselves. Some low-income families who would have liked to have a tutor simply couldn't afford one.

We hoped to remove these obstacles by having tutoring arrangements become an accepted part of 'early intervention programs' that treat deaf children from the time of diagnosis until three or four years of age. Just as these programs offer speech therapy lessons and auditory training sessions, they could also offer parents the opportunity to meet regularly with deaf adults who could show them how to improve communication with their child through Sign Language (Bouvet, 1979b). Introducing this language into programs for deaf children would in no way contradict efforts geared toward helping them speak vocally.

In 1979, however, not a single program was open to the project. It wasn't until 1981 that an early intervention program based on this bilingual approach was able to open with backing from the Ministry of Health.

In 1979, the only officially approved option available was to open a bilingual class for profoundly deaf children who, at six years old, were failing miserably in school. These children had undergone years of early intervention based on the most recognized methods, yet no system of linguistic communication had developed between them and their parents. Now that the children were also beginning to display behavioral problems — some of them serious — there was simply no place for them within existing educational structures. Since the conventional approach had failed these children, we were allowed to work with them according to our own approach.

We thus offered these older children the bilingual education we would have liked to undertake with newly diagnosed deaf infants and toddlers who could still be spared from ever having to experience failure in their attempts to communicate.

6 Opening a Bilingual Kindergarten Class for Deaf Children — 1979

In 1979 deaf individuals were not officially allowed to teach in schools as Sign Language instructors, yet there was no way we could set up a bilingual class without a deaf teacher. To begin the program, those in authority had to be convinced that visual speech and vocal speech were not antinomic but complementary speech modalities.

By September 1979, we were able to open a bilingual kindergarten class team-taught by a hearing and a deaf teacher (each of whom interacted with the children in her own language). Outlined below are the basic principles upon which the class was based.

The Underlying Principles and Goals of the Bilingual Class

Vocal language cannot truly be acquired without also learning Sign Language

Chapter 4 showed that sign languages are the only languages that allow deaf people to experience all the linguistic features of speech. Sign Language is thus *indispensible* if deaf children are to fully acquire language. This was the basic principle behind the bilingual class.

Sign Language allows deaf children to discover linguistic communication at the same age as hearing children who enjoy a positive learning environment. Being a visual language, Sign Language allows deaf children to *experience what a language is* without any limitations. This in turn gives them a better sense of what occurs in vocally produced verbal exchanges that all but escape them. In other words, if deaf children are given the opportunity to use a language they fully grasp, they can then understand *how vocal speech is used* even though they

141

cannot naturally acquire it. For this reason, learning Sign Language is absolutely fundamental to deaf children's acquisition of vocal speech. Among many observations to this effect, one mother made the following remark about her two-year-old son who had begun learning Sign Language: 'Now that he understands what a language is he is beginning to try to articulate words' (Thomas, 1979: 12).

Besides being the one language that can open all the doors of linguistic communication to deaf children, Sign Language is also the one language they can acquire *without delay*. As previously pointed out, deaf children of deaf parents speak gesturally at the same age that hearing children begin to speak vocally.

Children manipulate complex syntactic structures at a very young age — well before they acquire an abundant vocabulary, correct morphology or refined articulation. Wilder Penfield and Lamar Roberts, among others, have highlighted the importance of the 'biological clock of language learning' (Penfield & Roberts, 1959) and pointed out that the development of syntax marks a crucial point in language acquisition. As seen in Chapter 2, syntactic structures are rooted in the interactive processes that a mother and child begin to develop as soon as the child is born (Bruner, 1977). In other words, syntax emerges from a very specific learning process that will necessarily be unique for each and every child. It is hardly surprising then that differences in children's acquisition and command of language begin to surface at a very early age. In researching the nature of these differences, Lentin (1975) discovered a fact directly relevant to our work with deaf children: when three to four-year-old children have poorly developed syntax for their age, their rate of language learning tends to decrease rather than increase rapidly as it normally does in children of that age. In Lentin's words,

> If these syntactic articulations do not begin to function at the right moment (i. e. immediately following the child's first complete statements), language seems to remain 'poor' rather than function as it should; it revolves around a limited set of juxtaposed sentences with minimal subordination. Vocabulary continues to grow, and pronunciation and correct grammar progress to some degree, but language structures do not become more sophisticated, statements do not branch out, and the combinatorial does not become any richer. (Lentin, 1975: 91)

Lentin's studies thus corroborate those of Penfield and Roberts, showing that there exists a 'critical period' in the development of speech syntax. If children do not receive what they need *when they need it* to enrich their syntax, they can lose this potential altogether. In short, healthy language development hinges on respecting children's 'biological clock'.

Yet in vocal language, deaf children's biological clock cannot possibly be respected because it takes them years of hard work to grasp this language. Deaf children *can* gain command of syntactic structures at the right time (i. e. when they are very young), but only in Sign Language — a language they can fully perceive.

Learning English might be a luxury for a young French hearing child, but learning Sign Language is an *absolute necessity* for deaf children and must be an integral part of their education. Being the one language they can learn without delay if simply given the opportunity, Sign Language restores for deaf children one of the basic conditions of healthy language learning, namely accessing speech *at the right time* in terms of their development. Sign Language also fulfills all of the other basic conditions for language learning, as we shall now see.

Only Sign Language can reestablish for deaf children the natural conditions of language acquisition

Chapter 5 showed that a hearing mother can draw her deaf infant into language by talking to the child both in vocal words and in signs from Sign Language. By drawing on Sign Language, she allows her deaf infant to begin experiencing language through a *mother tongue*, just as other children do. Once put in contact with deaf adults, the child can then pick up Sign Language through natural language acquisition processes. That is, the child can benefit from words addressed to him or her in the *special child-directed speech register* and also from the *free-flowing speech* of an adult rambling on in the his or her presence without real concern for being understood. As we know, free-flowing speech is rich in affect and plays an important role in child language acquisition. This type of exchange is only possible, however, in a language fully accessible to the child. For a deaf child, that language is Sign Language.

Sign Language is also the one language in which deaf children have access to discourse spoken around them but not to them. Conversations in vocal language cut deaf children off from this extremely important language-learning situation because vocal language is imperceptible to deaf children unless the speaker addresses them directly and takes special care to make his speech 'visible'.

Sign Language is, in fact, the one language in which deaf children can benefit from all the various natural speech situations so vital to language acquisition. Similarly, it is the only language in which deaf children can *play with speech*.

In Sign Language, deaf children receive visual feedback from their own verbal activity and can enjoy *seeing* themselves speak just as hearing children enjoy *hearing* themselves speak. This allows deaf children to play with the material aspects of signifiers and to produce speech not meant to 'say' anything. Such word games play a fundamental role in the acquisition of language: 'Children learn to speak by playing with words' (Diatkine, 1976: 600).

In vocal language, such play is impossible. How can deaf children possibly enjoy playing with a language they have such difficulty even perceiving? How can they play with sounds they cannot hear?

This brings us to a final point. Because the nature of signs produced and signs received is identical in Sign Language (see page 104), it allows deaf children to identify with others in many different ways through speech itself. As we know, this process of identification is another important factor in language learning.

Through Sign Language, then, it is possible to restore for deaf children all the natural and indispensable conditions for language acquisition. Yet mere possibilities are not enough. Those conditions must be made a reality.

The use of Sign Language does not eliminate the need to nurture deaf children in linguistic communication

In our professional practice we have observed that once people understand that Sign Language opens the door to natural language acquisition in deaf children, they sometimes tend to believe that exposure to Sign Language is all deaf children need to learn language. But this is not the case at all.

Simply putting deaf children in contact with a fully accessible language does not eliminate all the work of language acquisition that must occur initially within communicative interactions with an adult.

Sign Language enables deaf children to acquire language 'naturally' in the same way that hearing children acquire vocal language. But these 'natural' learning processes still rely on an 'implicit pedagogy' that draws children into real 'learning situations'. As seen in Chapters 2 and 3, these situations cannot occur except under very particular 'luxury conditions' (Diatkine, 1975b).

Like all children, deaf children need to be tracked and guided in their linguistic development — even when this development occurs through Sign Language. If anything, the 'luxury conditions' of language acquisition are all the more imperative for deaf children because of the unique linguistic situation that deafness creates:

(1)   Deaf children are bound to become bilingual, regardless of whether their parents are deaf or hearing. But the experience of bilingualism will not be a positive one unless each language is acquired under healthy learning conditions.

(2)   Deaf children of hearing parents inevitably run into communication difficulties that gnaw at their verbal appetite. Unlike deaf children of deaf parents, those of hearing parents are not immersed in a sea of visual words exchanged with and around them right from the cradle. Greater attention must be given to drawing these children into speech — even if that speech is visual.

To summarize, affording deaf children a language they can acquire naturally does not eliminate their need for all the essential conditions of language acquisition. Deaf children need these conditions even more than other children do.

This fact has been sorely disregarded in recent years. Observations of deaf children communicating among themselves gesturally has led to the hasty conclusion that they must know how to speak their natural gestural language. When deaf children use gestures to communicate among themselves they are not speaking in Sign Language — a gestural language received from an *adult verbal model*. Most deaf children have never had an adult model. No efforts are made to help deaf children learn Sign Language; in fact, gestural communication is not even allowed in some of the educational establishments that receive them. Communication among deaf children certainly is based on gestures — some of which may come from Sign Language if by chance one of the children has deaf parents — but we must not assume that their gestures constitute a language. Children cannot learn a language simply through communicative interactions with other children. This is doubly true when the language in question is a stigmatized and forbidden one.

Yet the false conception that deaf children generally know Sign Language has nonetheless served as the basis for linguistic research. In attempting to compare the effectiveness of gestural and vocal communication, Pierre Oléron (1978) employed the following method:

A sender is presented with a stimulus that he is to describe through gestures. In the first five situations, the receiver has before him a set of objects that differ from each other in various characteristics. From among these objects, the receiver is to choose the one described by the sender. In the sixth situation, the stimulus is a model that the receiver must recreate by assembling the objects as described... The same experiment was conducted with hearing subjects expressing themselves orally... The sample deaf population was composed of 20 students from a specialized Parisian establishment,[1] and ranged in age from age 9; 11 to 15;4. They were divided into ten pairs of the same sex... The sample hearing population was composed of the same number of boys and girls, aged 15;0 to 17;8, from a CET[2] in the Paris region. They too were divided into ten pairs of the same sex... Communication was one-way: the receiver was not allowed to ask questions of the sender. (Oléron, 1978: 68, 80–81)

The results of the experiment led to the conclusion that gestural communication is not as effective as vocal communication.

Oléron acknowledges that he did not sufficiently control for the competency level of the deaf subjects in their gestural language. 'This competency could have been evaluated in a preliminary test' (ibid.: 80), he admits. He also concedes that the conditions under which the deaf subjects learned and practiced gestural language 'differed considerably from the conditions under which the hearing subjects learned and practiced oral language' (ibid.: 130). Nonetheless, Oléron does not call into question the basic validity of his conclusion that gestural communication is inferior to vocal communication. The fact is, however, the gestural and oral communication he observed merely reflected the varying verbal competency of the subjects sampled.

Other experiments, such as those of Loreli Bode (1974) and I. King-Jordan (1975), showed that when deaf subjects are selected according to their command of Sign Language (which they 'really' speak), Sign Language communication proves to be just as effective as vocal language communication. In his evaluation of these experiments, Grosjean (1979: 39) remarks that 'the opposite would be surprising'.

Children do not enter the world with a ready-made language in their hands if they are born deaf. Deaf children do not acquire Sign Language simply by not being forbidden to use gestural communication. As we have said, deaf children need the same very special learning conditions that hearing children do in order to acquire speech, even when this speech is visual-gestural and thus fully accessible to them.

The principles developed so far in this chapter provided the basis for our bilingual class. What then were the goals of this educational undertaking?

The goals of bilingual education for deaf children: normal language learning in an atmosphere of communication and success

Bilingualism is the only approach that affords deaf children a situation in which they can succeed in verbal communication. With Sign Language, deaf children do not experience any handicap in ensuring the success of their attempts to communicate, provided that in this language they have been offered the conditions necessary for language acquisition.

Sign Language restores for deaf children the atmosphere of easy communication children need to acquire language. It starts with what is positive in deaf children, namely their ability to express themselves in a visual mode. Upon this acknowledged strength, they are then offered the vocal speech they are missing. But this absence of vocal speech is not where teaching begins. First the children are recognized for who they are: complete language-inclined beings fully capable of satisfying their needs as speaking subjects in a visual mode. Deaf children can thus be received in the anticipation of their speech, just as other children are. As we know, this attitude of anticipation plays a fundamental role in speech acquisition.

In this way, we restored a normal language-learning situation in which the children learned to communicate and speak by communicating and speaking.

Similarly, one learns to succeed by succeeding. Our primary objective was to give deaf children the opportunity to experience successful verbal interaction so that they could come to enjoy and desire it. Once deaf children have experienced easily understanding others and making themselves understood in Sign Language, they realize what it means to speak. Consequently, they want to be able to interact verbally in *vocal language* as well, despite the great challenge it represents. They understand how vocal language is used even though their own perception and production of it remain patchy. In sum, this bilingual approach truly does draw deaf children into two different languages, each of which is equally valued in the classroom and at home.

Having set forth the principles and goals of our educational approach, we will now describe the class itself.

The Bilingual Class

The class was composed of five profoundly deaf children and one severely deaf child (see Appendix A for audiometric curves). There were two teachers — one deaf and one hearing (myself). The deaf teacher spoke in Sign Language and the hearing teacher in vocal language. Each language was thus embodied in a different person and presented independently of the other.

Before describing our classroom activities we must first introduce the children themselves.

The children and their families in terms of communication

In September 1979 five of the children were six years old and one was only four and a half. Their backgrounds were each different and unique,[3] but the one thing the five six-year-olds had in common when they joined the class was their utter failure at communication. This state of failure was seriously affecting their personalities. Some of them were prone to violent fits of anger and confrontational or unstable behaviors. Others tended to withdraw, appearing sad and abandoned, even absent. For some of the children, the clinical outlook was so bleak that they had already begun receiving psychological treatment. The clinical report on one of the children reads: 'sensitive, intelligent child, but presents psychological disorders probably as serious as his deafness'. So pronounced was this child's withdrawal that the school for deaf children where he had been placed could not keep him, and every other school his parents approached refused to accept him. Some of the children had also been diagnosed with 'associated disorders' in addition to their deafness. One had a tongue and lip coordination problem; another showed a degree of mental retardation.

It wasn't for lack of early treatment that these communication and behavioral problems had set in. Deafness had been diagnosed very early in each of these children (some at 9 months and some at 12). They had all immediately been fitted with a hearing aid and enrolled in vocal speech training. Yet not one of these children had been able to establish any kind of verbal communication with their parents.

By way of example, the following comments summarize the speech evaluation of one of the children upon enrollment in the class (she was 6;4 years old and had received four years of vocal speech training):

— does not talk; does not understand speech
— roughly articulates [f] [v] [p] and [t]; poor vowel sounds — opens mouth too wide;
— fleeting attention.

The five older children suffered serious attention problems. They made no eye-contact whatsoever with those seeking their attention. Yet these children must have experienced the importance of eye-contact in preverbal interactions with their mother when they were infants. This shows that when children cannot develop their communication skills, they tend to severely regress and even lose what communication skills they had acquired.

Our five six-year-old students had lost their foothold on communicative interaction and had been unable to enter into verbal dialogue. They therefore had no reason to maintain eye-contact, the purpose of which is to register the effect one has on others and to show that a response is expected. Loss of eye-contact can also be attributed to forced and unsuccessful vocal speech training. In the name of speech therapy, these children had been commanded to watch someone's lips in a very controlled environment that made any kind of meaningful interaction impossible. Diatkine (1980) notes that the deaf children he treats in his practice invariably seem to have been seriously violated through their eyes, and that this violation has made them lose their basic sense of curiosity and their interest in others. How can interaction be reestablished with these children who do not visually acknowledge their interlocutor? And isn't eye contact deaf children's primary means of making contact and communicating? For children who cannot hear the sounds of speech, losing the ability to interact visually is particularly serious.

Such was the condition of the five six-year-olds when they entered the class. Fortunately, this wasn't the case for the four and a half-year-old. Because of her age and other reasons we will later discuss, she had gone without communication for a shorter period of time.

Four of the children enrolled in September 1979. The other two joined the class in the following May, as the school year was coming to a close. However, we had been in frequent contact with the families of the two latecomers since November 1979, and since that time they had been familiarizing themselves with Sign Language in order to improve family communication.

This brings us to the families of these six children and what they thought bilingual education would do for their child. Agnès' (age 4;6) and Charles' (5;10) parents chose the bilingual class because they had recently learned that the deaf had a language. Agnès had been in vocal speech training since one year of age and Charles since the age of two, yet their parents had not been able to establish any kind of communication with them. Now they wanted to try Sign Language. They began attending classes offered once a week by the International Community for Visual Theater Research in Château de Vincennes. These classes were not particularly geared toward parents but intended for anyone interested in Sign Language. Because of this, the parents' motivations were somewhat different from their classmates', but the sessions did help them improve communication with their child.

When Agnès enrolled in the class, she had already been communicating with her family in signed French for one year and had been learning Sign Language with a deaf adult who visited weekly. Agnès knew that she was deaf. She had *active eye-contact* and had accumulated enough linguistic baggage to be able to understand and produce gestural statements such as, 'Tomorrow we are going to drive to the countryside'.

Charles' mother had started taking Sign Language classes shortly before he enrolled. In September 1979, the two of them had just begun to communicate. She managed to tell him little things about everyday matters such as, 'We are going to take the bus to school'; and Charles could produce statements composed of one or two signs, such as 'for Eva' (referring to a toy he wanted to give his friend Eva). But for a child of his age, these were very limited exchanges. Charles would react with extreme agitation, throw tantrums and avoid eye contact as a way of expressing his rage and dissatisfaction with this continually frustrating communication. Yet he hadn't lost the need to communicate.

Sabine's (6;4) and Rémi's (6;1) parents also chose the bilingual class because of the communication problems they were having with their child. But their choice did not come from a desire to enter deaf culture by becoming familiar with the language of the deaf. Since conventional methods had failed their child, they had no choice but to try an alternative route. They resigned themselves to trying what they thought of as 'the method that used gestures' because their child apparently couldn't do any better. In other words, these parents turned to the bilingual class not by choice but by process of elimination — their child had failed at everything else. Surely their child must have other disorders besides deafness, they thought. After all, other deaf children seemed to succeed where their child had failed. They didn't realize that their child's inability to communicate stemmed from an inappropriate pedagogy unsuited to his needs. These parents had been waiting years to be able to communicate with their child verbally, yet such communication never developed. In fact, family life had become so strained and unbearable that they had nearly ceased to show their child affection. Both Sabine and Rémi expressed their suffering in the only way they knew how — tantrums, impulsive behavior, provocation, withdrawal. And their parents, at wit's end, were reduced to treating them like extra-baggage that had to be dressed, fed and carted around, without being able to explain to them why these things were happening. In sum, these children had been steadily losing their status as speaking subjects, as partners with an active role to play in interaction.

Not surprisingly, both Sabine and Rémi arrived in class with very disturbed eye behaviors. Sabine's eyes rested on nothing and no one. They were devoid of expectation, empty and resigned. Rémi, on the other hand, was very attentive to objects but dodged other people's eyes with disconcerting regularity. His eyes darted away even before they could be met. On those rare occasions when his eyes did happen to meet others', they shouted defiance and provocation without a whisper of invitation.

We met Linda's and Patrick's parents in November. They had just found out that the deaf had a language and were beginning to explore new ways of relating with their deaf child. In both cases, family dynamics had become deeply disturbed, resembling those experienced in Sabine's and Rémi's families. Linda's parents contacted us after hearing our presentation on the bilingual class at a colloquium on deaf children. They had immediately recognized themselves in our description of the dynamics that develop between parents and children who are unable to establish any kind of verbal communication despite years of trying. They told Patrick's parents about the bilingual class and thus began a long process which eventually culminated with the enrollment of both children in our class the following May. Since Linda and Patrick had frequently changed schools and their parents had suffered considerable disappointments, both families were quite understandably hesitant to commit to a whole new educational program.

But neither parents hesitated to take Sign Language classes either in Château de Vincennes or at the Académie de la Langue des Signes located in the Saint-Jacques school. They also made arrangements to have the deaf teacher and one of the deaf interns from the bilingual class tutor their child in Sign Language. We were thus able to keep close tabs on each child's progress. Both children also participated in our Wednesday afternoon painting workshop.

When Linda and Patrick did join the class in May they already more or less belonged. By this time verbal communication had begun to develop between them and their parents. Yet they still had those hard-to-reach eyes and their behaviors contrasted starkly with those of the children we had already worked with for nine months.

Peering out from under his brow, Patrick would wait, his whole body tense with anxiety, ready to explode if disappointed by a response. Given the limited means by which he could communicate, it was very difficult for anyone to understand what he wanted. But at least Patrick still expected something from communication despite all the frustration it had caused him. Linda, on the other hand, did not interact at all. She would lower her head and refuse to look up.

The parents of these two children, like those of Charles and Agnès, knew that only bilingual education could meet their child's communication needs. And they realized that their child was not entirely at fault in their failure to communicate. Furthermore, since Sign Language had enabled these four children to begin communicating in little ways before joining the bilingual class, their parents knew that they were making the right educational choice. Rémi's and Sabine's parents would soon come to these same realizations.

This summarizes the communicative condition of the children and their parents at the outset of the bilingual class. The following section describes how the class was organized.

How the class was organized

During the first year, inadequate space in the available facilities made phys-ical arrangements less than ideal and prohibited us from teaching the children for more than two hours a day. Class could be held only from 3:00 to 5:00 in the afternoon in a classroom used from 9:00 to 2:45 for older children. The walls were reserved for the older children's materials and the furniture was hardly suited to kindergartners. But at least we had a place to meet — which was essen-tial — and a huge movable blackboard that could be brought down to the chil-dren's level.

We would push the large tables back against the walls, set chairs in a circle, and begin class.

Working with the children: storytelling with picture books. As the children sat cross-legged on their oversized chairs, we set about our primary task, which was to tell them stories. We told them real stories, like the ones children are always told from a tender age when all goes well (i. e. when the family atmosphere is a healthy one and a good relationship exists between the parents and their child). Every story was told twice — once by each of the teachers in her own language.

(1) Why tell stories to children who don't know how to speak? Telling stories to children who desperately need to learn to communicate, to understand speech and to express everyday matters, might seem like a waste of time. Why take such an approach with children who, for the most part, have never been told a story in their lives? Isn't this taking an incredible gamble? In our estimation, sto-rytelling was the one approach that would allow us to draw the children into speech while respecting the necessary conditions of language acquisition.

Many hearing children do not have anyone who takes the time to talk to them and tell them stories. Most of the words addressed to them are meant to 'scold and threaten' (Diatkine, 1975a: 13). These children do not receive their share of tirelessly told stories that would 'help them develop mental defenses against anxieties... For them, language is mainly a form of aggression...' (ibid.: 14). As we know, these are the children who eventually fail in school. They are unable to take interest in what is said to the class as a whole because they have never experienced the benefits and blessings of speech meant just for them in verbal interactions undertaken 'for the mere pleasure of it'. Since all teacher/student interaction is achieved through language, such children are unable to benefit from what school has to offer. It would seem that the role of kindergarten is to rescue such children from scholastic failure by allowing them to experience speech as a source of deep emotion and well-being.

This brings us back to the importance of pleasure and play in language acquisition. 'Teaching a child that verbal communication can be pleasurable is not an easy task', admits Diatkine (1975a: 14) in reference to hearing children. Yet this was the task before us, and it would be all the more difficult because the deaf children with whom we were working had suffered immensely in the area of communication itself.

The apparent uselessness and undemanding indulgence of our storytelling were precisely what guaranteed that our work with the children would be effective. This was the only way we could offer them language *as a gift* and thereby respect the conditions so essential to children in accessing speech. By using a visual language that made these conditions possible (see pages 143 and 144), we were providing the children with a language learning situation that came as close as possible to the natural language-learning process that normally begins at birth (see Chapter 2).

These deaf children had to be returned to their days of preverbal communication (see Chapter 2, page 39 and following). Like all children, they had known how to communicate preverbally but had then lost their momentum when that communication did not lead to speech. They also needed the chance to acquire verbal communication — something none of them had even begun to experience until quite recently (see Chapter 2, page 51 and following).

We realized that storytelling could create a very unique situation in which the children would able to return to and experience the various stages necessary to language acquisition.

Stories can draw deaf children back into extra-verbal dialogue. During the period of preverbal communication, a mother talks to her infant while interacting with him or her through multiple sensory channels. Her speech is part of the extra-verbal communication that occurs between her and her child through highly structured and ritualized activity sequences.

Such situations allow children to predict some of their mother's responses and thus enter into a preverbal dialogue that demonstrates intentionality and reciprocity. In this way, children become full partners in preverbal communication, and through that communication learn turn-taking. Since these first dialogues are always accompanied by the mother's speech, children are able to realize that speech is not so much a means of *conveying content* as a process of *entering into relationship*. This is how they come to the fundamental realization that, by its nature, speech is part of the connecting process and thus a vehicle of pleasure — the pleasure that comes with the satisfaction of one's need for communication and for companionship.

Through storytelling, we were able to recreate for the children all these characteristics of preverbal dialogue. Since they didn't yet know how to talk, our speech obviously far exceeded their verbal abilities, yet everything that enveloped our speech (i. e. our extra-verbal communication) was fully accessible to them. The telling of a story became a real ritual, a heterogeneous whole composed of facial expressions, body language, intonation, verbal rhythm, pauses, breathing patterns, gestures, etc. That exact ritual was repeated every time the story was told, and also repeated within the same telling if the story followed a repetitive format. In this way, we created situations in which the children were able to make predictions, just as a mother communicates with her infant. This ability gave the children the satisfaction of being able to *anticipate* a gesture, a face or a moment of suspense as the story unfolded. We then *responded* to their contributions, letting them see how happy we were to be able to understand them, and giving them the pleasure of feeling understood. Such interactions created an atmosphere of well-being that also fulfilled our own need to be able to anticipate the children's communicative abilities. The children thus experienced themselves in a positive light. They knew that they more than lived up to our expectations every time they were able to anticipate what would happen next. Feeling important in our eyes, they reclaimed their status as *active partners* in dialogue, which was very important for these children who had never been able to live up to their parents' vocal speech expectations and too often had felt like a disappointment and a failure in others' eyes. As we know, self-esteem and positive self-image play an important role in child development, and the only way that children can gain such confidence is by experiencing successful interaction with others.

Storytelling thus restored the children to their role as active partners in dialogue through extra-verbal communication. In rediscovering the pleasures of preverbal interaction, they also rediscovered the pleasures of *eye-contact*. Because we offered them the opportunity to succeed, they followed us with their eyes, willingly looking at us to share in the pleasures of a well-being established through extra-verbal communication. Since this dialogue included verbal communication, the children came to realize that speech was part of the *connecting process*, and thus a vehicle of pleasure.

In short, the children found themselves in a situation that allowed them to access speech in the same way that all children do — through successful preverbal interaction.

By introducing the children to extra-verbal communication, we also drew them into speech. This process paralleled the one described earlier in our definition of a *mother tongue*. In restored dialogue, the children expressed themselves in their own individual ways, and we responded with speech that matched their expectations.

Stories can introduce deaf children to language through the special child-directed speech register. Once the children regained pleasure in eye-contact and extra-verbal communication, they were well on their way to acquiring speech and were ready to soak up the words with which our stories were told. These words were always based on picture books and had all the characteristics of the special register used with children who do not yet know how to talk.

The children loved to look at the pictures in the storybooks we shared with them. Deaf children are keenly curious about books and illustrations because normally they are deprived of communication and verbal explanations in an educational system that does not know how to provide them. Two-dimensional representations of three-dimensional objects allow deaf children to understand the arbitrary nature of representation. Using those representations, they develop the ability to arrange things in series and categories. In searching for picture-book representations of familiar objects they become attentive to size, form and color. In short, picture books help deaf children to discover and better understand reality.

Because the children were attentive to illustrations in the stories we told them, they were able to understand the essence of what was being said. For example, when we said, 'The wolf knocks at the door: knock! knock!' while showing the children an illustration of a wolf knocking at a door, they had all of the situational elements they needed to understand what was being said. Our speech thus maintained the *semantic characteristics* of the child-directed speech register in that it expressed the here-and-now of the exchange situation in such a way that the children could deduce the meaning of what was said from what they saw.

Storytelling also nicely accommodated all of the *phonological characteristics* of the child-directed speech register. To make our words easy for the children to perceive, we spoke slowly and with increased intonation. Such accentuation added greater definition to divisions between and within sentences and even served to highlight particular units right down to the word. As discussed earlier, the iconicity of Sign Language can be highlighted or obscured in many ways depending on the discourse situation (see page 101). So enhanced is this iconicity in child-directed speech that a uninformed observer watching the deaf teacher tell the class a story might think that she was resorting to mime — not using a real language. But the deaf teacher did speak in Sign Language, but at a slower rhythm and with greater intonation. Such devices make the *translucency* of certain units readily apparent. That is, the connection between the sign and what it represents becomes immediately obvious provided that the content is already understood. Such was the case in our storytelling with picture books because the illustrations clearly revealed the content of the story.

We made it easy for the children to follow visual speech by rendering it as 'translucent' as possible, specifically relating it to the situation at hand and producing it in such a way that the iconicity of the signs became apparent. With such attention given to signifiers themselves, the children began to appreciate the *poetic dimension* of speech and to appropriate it for the pleasure of its physical qualities. In Sign Language, this pleasure might be associated with the particular movements, handshapes or rhythm of a sentence, and in vocal language, with the flow of face and lip movements. The children became aware of speech as a *physical reality* through the phonological features of the child-directed speech register, and they acquired it because it was physically fun to manipulate.

Storytelling also preserved the *discursive qualities* of this special register by offering children repetitive and situational 'verbal episodes'. The children particularly liked stories in which nearly identical episodes were repeated again and again. *The Three Little Pigs* was one such a favorite. Each little pig encounters someone who can sell him material to build a house, and each encounter involves a very similar verbal episode. When the wolf enters the story, three more very similar episodes ensue. Virtually the same dialogue occurs as the wolf tries to enter each little pig's house. Such repetition enabled the children to *predict* what would happen next and to better understand the storyline. Consequently, they 'focused increasingly on the verbal formation' (Lentin, 1975: 172) of the story as it was told and retold with all the discursive qualities of the child-directed speech register. This highly ritualized process made the story predictable. Much of the charm storytelling held for the children seemed to lie in their knowledge that a tale could be retold as many times as they wished.

Finally, storytelling matched the *syntactic qualities* of the child-directed speech register, which does not call for syntactic simplicity, but for a manner of speaking that helps children develop strategies for acquiring the syntactic structures inherent in any utterance. On average, interrogatives and imperatives are much more frequent in child-directed speech than in adult speech. The same was true of our storytelling because of all the dialogue between characters. Also, a story cannot be told without coordinating conjunctions (e.g. but, or), subordinating conjunctions (e.g. because, if, when) and relative pronouns (e.g. who, that). The children acquired such syntax by hearing it used again and again in the verbal episodes of the stories we told. The story in which a puppy searches for a lost little girl by asking various animals if they have seen her illustrates this point. Each episode ends with a 'but' sentence like, 'But the snail hadn't seen her...'.

In sum, storytelling enabled us to introduce the children to speech in exactly the same way that other children are, that is, through natural interactions having all the characteristics of the child-directed speech register. By telling the children stories, we recreated for them the natural situations through which language is learned — one of which is storytelling itself.

(2) Which stories should be told? Satisfying stories that help give meaning to life. Each of the children in our class had been seriously deprived of communication until relatively late in his or her life. Such deprivation may even have robbed them of their need for interaction and rendered them unable to communicate effectively through speech or all that envelops speech (cf. eye behaviors, under the heading 'The children and their families in terms of communication', earlier in this chapter). Unbearably frustrated in relating to others, their lives had sunk into chaos. Our goal was to draw them out of their suffering into the well-being that comes from connecting with others in positive ways.

More importantly than teaching the children to speak, we sought to nourish their personal lives and thereby enrich their interactions. We told the children fairy tales because these were stories that could help them find meaning in life and develop psychologically. Bettelheim (1975: 25) explains: 'The fairy tale's concern is not useful information about the external world, but the inner processes taking place in an individual'. By externalizing these internal processes in the form of simple, straightforward characters and clear-cut scenarios, fairy tales help children know themselves; they also subtly suggest how to resolve difficulties and enjoy a better life. Fairy tales do not impose anything; they let children choose what is meaningful to them. But fairy tales always bring promise of a happy ending regardless of what may befall the hero; they offer the 'assurance that one can succeed' (Bettelheim, 1975: 10). For the children in our class, this was an important message. These children had experienced failure all too often and had led extremely difficult lives, tossed about in a world they couldn't possibly understand for lack of communication and humanizing words. As Dolto (1977: 25) explains, 'All that is not spoken remains foreign, not something children can relate to'. The difficulty (or impossibility) of understanding others and making oneself understood had caused the children in our class immense frustration. For this reason, we especially tried to tell them stories that might echo their own emotions and thus make them feel understood. The fairy tale 'takes these existential anxieties and dilemmas very seriously and addresses itself directly to them: the need to be loved and the fear that one is thought worthless; the love of life, and the fear of death' (Bettelheim, 1975: 10).

What Bettelheim says about the value of fairy tales for 'modern' children also applies to deaf children:

The fairy-tale hero proceeds for a time in isolation, as the modern child often feels isolated. The hero is helped by being in touch with primitive things — a tree, an animal, nature — as the child feels more in touch with those things than most adults do. The fate of these heroes convinces the child that, like them, he may feel outcast and abandoned in the world, groping in the dark, but, like them, in the course of his life he will be guided step by step, and given help when it is needed. Today, even more than in past times, the child needs the reassurance offered by the image of *the isolated man who nevertheless is capable of achieving meaningful and rewarding relations*[4] with the world around him. (Bettelheim, 1975: 11)

Our storytelling approach can thus be summarized as follows. First we drew the children back into extra-verbal dialogue, where they realized that 'statements', by their very nature, are a way of being together, a connecting process. From there we brought them to realize that 'statements' also open up a whole new world that can help them sort out their emotions and their need to interact and relate.

To speak is to come into one's own individuality (see pp. 16–32). But children can hardly acquire speech if they haven't experienced situations that allow them to gain a sense of who they are and where they stand.

We speak to make things different from what they are, to transform want into the pleasure of desire. In this way we avoid succumbing to the ache of want or 'the pain of desire' (Diatkine *et al.*, 1977: 119). Yet before children can undertake this transformation, they must have a sense of themselves and have faced their wants.

The children in our class had experienced so much conflict in their lives that they had reached the point of succumbing to the pain of their desires, which would have become bearable had they been shaped into words. Fairy tales offered these children a world where they could be emotionally nourished and restored. Fairy tales also brought order and meaning to their lives and revived their sense of expectation — long ago abandoned in the maze of their struggles and unanswered questions.

Within the vast array of children's stories, distinguishing those that qualify as fairy tales can be difficult. The criteria we adopted were those set forth by Bettelheim. First, the story had to have a happy ending; and second, the characters and events had to be straightforward so that, through easy identification with them, children could find meaning in their lives and discover speech that they could recreate and reinvent. To use an expression from the dedication of Lewis Carroll's *Through the Looking Glass* (1939: 166), we chose stories that the children could accept as a 'love-gift'.

We also considered the illustrations of a story. We looked for books with readily meaningful and pleasing images. We did not choose books based on vocabulary but on content. Children do not learn to speak from lists of words but from situational utterances that they want to receive and produce. People who came to observe the class often asked how we went about 'building vocabulary'. We didn't. Research by André Tabouret-Keller (1970) on children's lexicons shows that a good deal of their vocabulary (54–71%) does not correspond to the 1,034 words considered basic French (Tabouret-Keller, 1970: 100). 'The lexicon of children', explains Frédéric François (1978: 110), 'is not composed of common vocabulary but of vocabulary specific to certain characteristic exchange situations'. Children learn to speak by being spoken to about things that touch and interest them. Fairy tales are a magnificent means of creating such interaction. But the magic is in the *telling* of a tale; a child's experience of a story largely depends on how it is told.

(3) How to tell a story. Mothers and fathers can make good storytellers when they know and relate well to their child. This was not the case for us as teachers. We found ourselves facing not one, but several children with whom it was difficult to establish relations.

Consequently, we had to work on each fairy tale in advance, learning to tell it in a way that would make the children want to pay attention and follow along. This preparation required the joint effort of both teachers because we would each be telling the children the same story in our own language. All the same detail, repetition and emotion had to be present in both languages so the children would recognize the story as the same in both versions.

The first step in jointly preparing a story was to choose one that met the criteria described above and was pleasing to both teachers. To achieve real sharing and interaction, the children needed to sense that the adult storyteller was also enjoying the story. Since the children's enthusiasm often heightened the storyteller's own pleasure, the story embodied greater enjoyment and well-being every time it was told — all to the children's increasing delight.

Once we chose a story we both liked, we would prepare a short and simple version based on the story's illustrations. We did not actually *read* the fairy tales because text in children's books does not resemble *situation-based speech* and does not adhere to the criteria of the child-directed speech register. Take, for example, the following written text:

...But it seemed as though the land where he [the bear] had arrived was deserted: not a single house, not a single animal. Nothing but snow and forest.

We would transform this text into an oral utterance reflecting what was depicted in the accompanying illustration: 'The bear comes to a forest. There is no house, no animal. The bear sees only snow, lots of snow, and trees, lots of trees'.

While not taking away from the substance of the story, we did not hesitate to simplify it and drop a few details here and there in order to keep the story well within the children's attention span.

Preferably, each teacher learned the story by heart so that she could make it come to life and not have to fumble for words or what came next. By knowing the story backwards and forwards, we were able to turn our attention to the children's reactions and adjust our rhythm accordingly. Knowing a story well also freed us to play with signifiers and concentrate on the materiality of our speech to highlight its *poetic features*, which the children drank in. As a result, what began as the storyteller's story ended up as a tale told in unison — something that belonged much more to the children than it did to the storyteller.

The more we liked a story and the better we each knew how to tell it, the more attentive we could be to the children's reactions. We would notice them cling to one detail but not another, savor a particular word for its feel, or echo a dialogue with much greater emphasis than we ourselves would have given it.

The 'translucency' of Sign Language, as spoken in a poetic register, helped the children to enter into the fairy tales. Not surprisingly, they learned the Sign Language version of the stories much more quickly than the vocal version. But since they found the same feeling conveyed in both, they avidly followed the hearing teacher's words even though her expressive faces and lip movements were all they could emulate. In short, they discovered that vocal speech was a vehicle of pleasure, too.

In addition to identifying with the characters and events presented in stories, the children also identified with the adults who told them. More specifically, the children identified with and imitated the way the storytellers spoke in Sign Language and in vocal language respectively. The children gradually became attentive to vocal speech even though their deafness prevented them from appropriating all of its qualities. They started translating the hearing teacher's stories into Sign Language as they followed along through speechreading. Sometimes they even got ahead of her, anticipating in sign what was coming next.

In this way, real interaction developed between the children and the two adults who tirelessly told them stories over and over again. We carefully prepared and rehearsed these stories for the children, but it was their touch that refined them.

We did not offer the children any explanations as to the significance of a fairy tale since, as Bettelheim (1975) points out:

> Adult interpretations, as correct as they may be, rob the child of the opportunity to feel that he, on his own, through repeated hearing and ruminating about the story, has coped successfully with a difficult situation...we find meaning in life...by having understood and solved personal problems on our own, not by having them explained to us by others. (Bettelheim, 1975: 18–19)

As we lived the telling of a fairy tale together, the children rediscovered the pleasures of watching their interlocutor. We observed them each latch on to different words and expressions depending on their individual desires, needs and identifications. They did not receive 'the image of a speech which had a structure even before it came into existence' (Barthes, 1967: 19) but the image of a speech to be discovered and made one's own.

Storytelling engaged the children in metalinguistic activities. It made them wonder about 'statements', which they now saw as objects to be analyzed and studied.

(4) Stories became the basis for speech activities. Once the children discovered how enjoyable verbal interaction could be, they wanted to speak as we did. They wanted to take this speech, full of promise for their personal well-being, and make it their own. They would repeat a sign or part of a statement in Sign Language and, just for fun, label what they saw in illustrations. We let them know we understood by repeating what they had said. The resulting dialogue thus revolved around the children's own 'statements'. Since each of their attempts to express something was affirmed by an adult who offered a correct form of their 'statement' in return, they experienced the pleasure of *being understood*. In short, we reestablished for the children the fundamental processes of child speech acquisition. Such 'statement'-focused interactions represented the children's first *metalinguistic* activity. They occurred first in Sign Language, the language in which deaf children do not experience any limitations. We must point out, in this regard, that nothing could substitute for the deaf teacher, who understood the children's 'statements' better than any hearing person ever could. It was through Sign Language that the children first entered into language, and only a deaf person could thoroughly understand their verbalizations and thereby guarantee them the feedback they needed.

It wasn't long, however, before the children made attempts at verbal expression in vocal language as well. Here and there a child would make a lip movement in reference to a picture. These were labels the hearing teacher could correctly repeat for the children, thereby giving them the pleasure of being understood even when attempting something as difficult as vocal speech.

Affirmed in their attempts to speak in Sign Language and in vocal language, the children came to identify with both teachers — deaf and hearing.

Storytelling thus served as the basis for a series of metalinguistic activities in oral language (spoken in the presence of interlocutors) that drew the children into speech. Storytelling also drew them into written language. The children quickly became aware of the written text that accompanied each picture in story books. If, in telling a story, we happened to skip a few pages, the children would call it to our attention, pointing not to the skipped pictures but to the skipped text, and insisting that there was some writing for which we had not accounted. Thus, parallel to becoming interested in *oral language* in the two languages we offered them, the children also developed an interest in *written language*. In response to their interest in both aspects of language, we would write short sentences for them on the blackboard.

Introduction to writing. The sentences we selected to write on the blackboard were those that the children liked best in a story, either for their form or their content. For instance, on 26 October 1979, we wrote out these sentences from the book *Les bons amis* (Album du Pére Castor, Flamarion):

Le lapin a faim, il trouve deux carottes.
(The rabbit is hungry; he finds two carrots.)

Le cheval n'est pas là!
(The horse isn't there!)

In French Sign Language, the children liked the words LAPIN and CHEVAL which have the same placement but a different movement and handshape. When one knows the meaning of these signs, their form clearly evokes the animals they represent, which delights animal-loving children. The relative translucency of the signs FAIM and TROUVE also pleased the children. The sign PAS LA does not evoke its content at all, but the rhythm of it grabbed the children's attention; in the context of the story, it was a sign full of emotion — the rabbit was disappointed to find that the horse wasn't home.

In vocal French, the children liked how the words *lapin*, *pas là* and *faim* were formed — all of them are easy to see on the lips and thus easy to imitate. Also, the children were intrigued with the fact that *lapin* and *pas là* form a mirror image of each other (they are composed of the same two lip formations but in reverse order).

Here are a few more examples of sentences written on the blackboard. Those we presented on 19th May 1980, came from the fairy tale *Le roi, la reine et l'enfant* (*Belles histoires de pomme d'Api*, Ed. Bayard):

Le roi et la reine n'ont pas d'enfants.
(The king and queen have no children.)

Ils vont chercher un enfant dans la maison rose.
(They go looking for a child in the pink house.)

Il faut trouver la clef pour ouvrir la porte.
(They must find the key to open the door.)

We offered the children these sentences *as a gift*, as a response to their curiosity about written text. Delighted by the regularity and fixed nature of the written word, they often searched through the storybook to find the exact words we had written on the board.

With the blackboard between us, each teacher presented the sentences to the children in her own language. The deaf teacher said the sentences in Sign Language first, showing how each sign corresponded to certain written words or phrases. (As explained earlier, no one-to-one correspondence exists between the two languages. Through morphological variations, a single sign can incorporate what separate grammatical words express in vocal languages.) When the deaf teacher finished, the hearing teacher would then say the sentences out loud, showing the children how her lip movements corresponded to each of the written words. (Here there was a word-for-word correspondence since what was written and what was said belonged to the same language.)

Besides satisfying the children's curiosity about writing, this activity was cause for repeating those sentences the children liked best. In other words, it established one of the *discursive* characteristics unique to child-directed speech: ample repetition.

Using these sentences, the children engaged wholeheartedly in matching oral statements with their written representation. The deaf teacher would say a sentence in Sign Language and have one of the children point out the corresponding written sentence on the blackboard. The children never tired of matching Sign Language statements (which they knew by heart and loved to see again and again) with sentences written on the blackboard. The exercise was then repeated with the hearing teacher giving the statements in vocal language. After paying close attention to her face and the way her lips moved, the children would go to the blackboard and indicate the written sentence that matched what they saw on her lips. As an aid, the hearing teacher used gestures developed by Suzanne Borel-Maisonny that clearly evoke the articulatory and written characteristics of each phoneme. In addition to helping the children memorize how different sounds were represented in writing, these gestures also aided them in physically producing the phonemes and recognizing them visually on the lips. Once the children could easily recognize each of the sentences with the aid of these gestures, the hearing teacher then repeated them without the gestures. The children thus came to recognize speech through speechreading alone.

Since the children were eager to surpass what was asked of them, they quickly mastered these *recognition exercises* and moved ahead, trying to *read on their own*. In this *evocation exercise*, they attempted to produce in Sign Language and in vocal language the sentences they saw in written form. Delighted by this new-found ability, they soon uttered short, well-formed statements in each language.

Once the children became comfortable with reproducing written sentences verbally, they were eager to perform *memory exercises* by assuming the teacher's role. They would produce a statement and ask a classmate to come to the board and point out the corresponding written sentence. This truly was a memory exercise because the children did not want to give away the answer by letting the other children see them read the sentence they were going to produce. It was not until December 1980, after a year and three months of recognition and reproduction exercises, that they engaged in this memory exercise. They did so first in Sign Language but in no time at all they spontaneously began memorizing sentences in vocal language as well, even though this was much more demanding.

In sum, the pedagogical environment we established through storytelling with picture books simultaneously drew the children into oral and written language. They quickly understood that writing was a language too, and sought to understand the written words they saw in the stories we told them. For deaf children, written words have the added benefit of being fully accessible through sight alone, unlike vocally produced oral words. In becoming intrigued with written language, the children quickly grasped its various uses. They also knew that writing held the key to storytelling and was thus a source of pleasure. They wanted to learn written language because they sensed the possibilities it could open up for acquiring knowledge on one's own without depending on an interlocutor.

The children often saw us writing because we regularly jotted down observations throughout class. When they questioned us about our notes, we explained what they were for. In this way, the children came to understand writing as a *memory tool*. We also involved them in our written correspondence with their parents; they thus came to appreciate writing for its function in *long-distance communication*. Little by little they grasped all the inherent functions of written language. It's not that we emphasized written language over oral language; we showed the unique properties and purposes of each. A healthy upbringing in our society, brings children into contact with both modes of linguistic communication right from birth. As Foucambert (1976: 62) writes: 'Like speech, reading is an affective and relational element of the environment in which children live ...children learn to read because they live in a world of written communication...'. This was the same environment we hoped to create in our bilingual class.

While offering the children *oral communication* in two languages, one of which let them fully experience *what it means to speak*, we simultaneously gave them the opportunity to discover *written language* and *what it means to write*.

Through playing with two languages in activities centered around written representations of vocal language, the children came to realize that language was in itself an *object of knowledge*. Children need this awareness not only to acquire written language, but also to learn to speak. As Jakobson (1960: 356) notes, 'Any process of language learning, in particular child acquisition of the mother tongue, makes wide use of such metalingual operations'.

In the process of wondering about writing and its correspondence to oral language, the children were actively acquiring the latter; this curiosity is what led to oral–verbal interplays of questions and answers about the stories.

Asking questions about the stories. If we told the story about a little black rooster who finds a gold coin, there would be no sense in asking the color of the rooster or the coin. Clearly, the answers to these questions are already known, and questions are asked to find out something one doesn't know. But such questions would be meaningful if they were part of a *game* and satisfied the children's need to play with language and to manipulate it solely for the fun of discovering how it works.

We had to wait until the children had gained metalinguistic perspective on their words before we could engage them in such question and answer games about the stories. Within two weeks of the first day of class in September 1979, the children had begun to make metalinguistic associations between oral and written language. Yet it was a full three months before they were ready to engage in the utterly gratuitous metalinguistic activity of playing with questions solely as an opportunity to make statements.

Grasping the *meaning of questions* was not easy for these deaf children who had gone without linguistic communication for so long. Having been unrecognized as speaking subjects, they were not accustomed to being asked questions. Through the *metalinguistic* activity of being asked questions about stories, however, they gradually came to comprehend how questions function.

We believe our approach paralleled how children naturally come to understand the meaning of questions. Mothers ask their infant questions to which they both know the answer. For instance, a mother will ask her child the color of something right in front of them. In this way, she gives her child the satisfaction of showing what he or she *knows about language*. Mothers introduce their child to the meaning of questions through all sorts of metalinguistic language manipulation. We did the same with the children in our class. They loved question and answer games because such games gave them the chance to show what they knew about language. But question and answer games were possible only because the children had already become capable of relating to speech metalingually. Unfortunately, educators of deaf children often neglect to follow this step-by-step process. They present question-and-answer type language exercises before the children know how to play with speech and· sometimes even before they have rediscovered the meaning of dialogue or become active partners in interaction.

Storytelling provided the metalinguistic atmosphere that brought forth the children's first spontaneous verbal expressions, that is, speech meant *to say something*.

(5) Stories also became the basis for the children's spontaneous verbalizations. Once the children entered into extra-verbal dialogue and began playing with verbal units during storytelling, they also began speaking up. In fact their first spontaneous verbal utterances came from the stories themselves. The children took words they had played with in storytelling activities and used them for their own purposes. Just fifteen days after Sabine was first exposed to Sign Language, she *spoke spontaneously*, deliberately using the signs MEAN and RED. These two signs were very prominent in the first story she had been told — a story that she constantly asked us to repeat throughout the first quarter. It was about some mean tigers who want to eat a little black boy. The first tiger spares him his life in exchange for his red vest. Each tiger does likewise in exchange for the boy's blue pants, green umbrella and pink shoes. In the end, the little boy recovers all his clothes and returns home very happy. Incidentally, this is the same story that prompted Sabine to begin learning the names of colors — which she then taught her mother in Sign Language.

On 7th March 1980 Rémi (another child who began without any exposure to Sign Language and no language of his own) said to Charles, who was being punished, '*Je me moque de toi*'. Rémi had acquired this expression a month earlier when we told the story of *The Ugly Duckling* who was mocked by other animals because he looked so different.

Quite clearly, it was because the children had been nourished with storytelling that they began to speak. Once they did, we set aside time for each of them to speak and express themselves.

This brings us to describing how class time was structured around the above mentioned activities.

(6) The division of class time during the first quarter of the 1980–81 school year. As detailed above, storytelling led to various related activities. These activities led to a structured and ritualized classroom routine which, in the Fall of 1980, included the seven following periods:

(i) Welcome time. Once we had established linguistic communication, the children always seemed to arrive to class with something to say. One might tell us he left his glasses at home, another that someone spilled noodles on his head in the cafeteria, etc. These were instances of authentic child-adult conversation. After the Easter vacation, 1980, we started to set aside a longer welcome time on Mondays so that each child could have a chance to tell what he or she had done on Sunday. By this time, some of the children were even able to recount their entire weekend.

(ii) Storytelling time. For more than a year, the deaf teacher always had the honor of telling a story first since it was easier for the children to become engaged in the story through Sign Language. But starting in mid-October 1980, the activity began with the hearing teacher so the children could hear stories first in vocal language (with which they were becoming familiar). A story was told first in Sign Language only when presented for the very first time.

(iii) Question time. Questions about the stories were still first asked in Sign Language and then in vocal language. The children had become fairly comfortable with questions in Sign Language, but remained uneasy with them in vocal language. Thus we preferred to continue introducing this activity in Sign Language, which was easiest for the children, so they could then rely on mental guesswork when asked the same questions vocally. As discussed earlier, speechreading allows a person to recognize what he or she expects to perceive, but not what remains to be discovered or understood. By asking questions in Sign Language first, we prepared the children for what they would perceive through speechreading.

(iv) Reading time: recognizing a few story-excerpted sentences on the blackboard. The children would come to the blackboard and point out the written sentence that corresponded to the statement they were given in Sign Language or vocal language. We selected those sentences the children seemed to like the best during the story either because of the physical qualities of the signifiers or because of their content (see page 162). The children really enjoyed this reading exercise (begun in October 1979) and could do it well in both languages. Thus, we could easily begin the exercise in vocal language.

(v) Reading time: reproducing and memorizing the sentences. On their own initiative, the children started trying to read sentences on the blackboard and to provide the corresponding oral statement for each teacher in her own language. From there, they memorized how to produce the sentences both vocally and gesturally.

(vi) Writing time: learning writing patterns. Writing intrigued the children right from the start and they soon wanted to learn how. We thus had them

practice writing *whole words* in cursive handwriting. We purposely did not begin with isolated letters. Writing involves mastering a linear pattern, and no such pattern becomes apparent except when letters are joined together to form whole words. We would select words from that day's story and write them out in large writing on the blackboard. The children came up and traced it several times with their finger in order to grasp the flow of the pattern. Without referring to the model, they then tried to write the words themselves, the only rule being that they weren't allowed to lift the chalk from the board in the middle of a word (this would interrupt the flow of the pattern). If they couldn't do it, they would go back to the model and trace it some more with their finger. In this way, each child learned the patterns of written words at his or her own pace.

(For reading exercises, we printed rather than hand-wrote sentences on the board. Printing was easier for the children to decipher and corresponded graphically to text they found in storybooks.)

(vii) Free time. Before class let out, we always gave the children a little free time when they could do as they pleased. Often they would go to the library corner, pick out a favorite book and ask the deaf teacher to read it to them again. They often insisted that the hearing teacher come over and follow along. In sum, the children would recreate, of their own initiative, the setting we always provided in which both teachers told them the same story. Some of the children even took advantage of free time to read by themselves. They would choose a book and enjoy recognizing certain words and sentences — which they would translate to themselves in Sign Language.

This free time was also very important to us as teachers. It allowed us to observe the children returning to particular activities and inventing new ones of their own. Such observations enabled us to better respond to the children's desires relative to oral and written language.

The seven activities that defined the bilingual class during the Fall of 1980 had evolved from storytelling alone (begun in September 1979) and reflected our growing interaction with the children. Likewise, these particular activities contained their own seeds of transformation. Our description of class activities during a particular time period is not meant to serve as a definitive teaching model — the activities themselves are continually evolving. Our purpose is to show how these activities all developed around storytelling, which itself was the basis for the children's acquisition of Sign Language and vocal language, in both its oral and written form.

As described above, these storytelling activities took place in both languages, one after the other. We always began in Sign Language until the children could accomplish the activity equally well in both; then we would begin in vocal language.

At some point during the class period, each child was taken aside for a personal speech therapy session. Since the children understood what speech was about and could approach language metalingually, they enjoyed their speech training sessions and took real pleasure in actively participating. The children were particularly eager to practice producing sentences in vocal language because they were always drawn from the story told in class.

When class was over, the children did not necessarily want to leave. Instead of going to get their coats they would go get a book or start writing on the blackboard even though they had just spent three intense hours in such activities. (Starting in September 1980, we were able to hold class during the more regular school hours of 1:30 to 4:30 instead of 3:00 to 5:00.)

This completes our description of how we worked with the children. Next we will explain how we worked with their parents.

Working with parents: Helping them see their deaf child as a person who speaks

Our work with the children could not be fully effective without real cooperation from their parents. Aren't parents primarily responsible for introducing their child to speech? Are they not their children's first language teachers? Unfortunately, the parents of the children in our class had been so deprived of this role that they had practically given up trying to interact with their child, whom they could no longer recognize as a speaking being. Addressing other parents, one couple with a deaf child writes:

> Have you noticed how little contact you have with your deaf child and how accustomed you've become to that fact? For us, it took only two weeks of Sign Language to realize with dismay how fully we had settled into not communicating with Ariane except, of course, in very vague ways or by being affectionate with her... How much had been left unsaid because there was no way to say it! (Meyer & Meyer, 1980: 21)

Our role was to help the parents restore dialogue with their deaf child. Sign Language came as a great relief to them in their efforts to interact with their child. By accompanying their vocal words with signs from Sign Language, they were finally able to verbally communicate effectively and with relative ease.

As part of the bilingual class, the deaf teacher held Sign Language class once a week for the children's parents. No vocal language was used in these classes. If a sign was not understood, the teacher would explain its meaning through mime and extra-verbal communication. This was very important in that it gave the parents the opportunity to better understand visual communication and allowed them to experience their deaf child's situation. It also let them discover what rich communication could occur solely through the visual channel. The parents came to realize that, in his or her own way, their child was a speaking being, too. The teacher also took advantage of class time to brief the parents on the story currently being told to the children. This enabled the parents to tell their child the story, too, or at least understand it if their child tried to tell it to them. And the parents used class time to ask the deaf teacher how to say various expressions they constantly needed to communicate with their child. For instance, they asked for link words like 'because', 'if' or 'when', signs for various family relations, and basic everyday vocabulary. On occasion they also asked the meaning of an unfamiliar sign they saw their child use.

The class was open not just to the children's parents but to any close relation who wanted to be able to communicate with the children — a grandmother, an aunt, a sibling. The older sister of one child attended regularly and became a great help to her parents. (It is easier to learn a new language as an 11-year-old than as an adult.)

We noticed that some parents learned faster than others. Some quickly amassed a nice core of signs while others needed more time. But the Sign Language class effectively helped all of them to improve communication with their child.

The class also gave the parents a chance to have regular contact with a deaf person. This was very beneficial since it helped them better comprehend the realities their child's life.

Two of the children's parents had never met a deaf adult or seen Sign Language before coming to this class. As the weeks went by, their faces became more relaxed and their fingers began to move. We also noticed that these parents were getting to know their child better now that they had begun talking with him or her through signed French.

Without exception, all the parents found they needed to supplement their weekly Sign Language class with a private class at home, which required finding and paying for a deaf tutor. The advantage of this arrangement was that it provided the deaf children with a deaf model at home in the heart of their family and helped them feel that their parents had really accepted them as different.

The group class for parents lasted for a good hour and was followed by a meeting with both the deaf and hearing teacher. We informed each other on communication in the classroom and at home. One mother realized, for example, that she never gave her daughter the opportunity to make her own choices — what dessert to eat, what clothes to wear. Yet these were the situations most conducive to dialogue.

The parents offered each other real support in learning to approach their deaf child as having the same need for interaction as other children. They also shared the changes that occurred in their relationship with their child once verbal communication was established: the tantrums had died down and a tenderness had developed; a boy had become affectionate; a girl had kissed her parents for the first time. In short, they told of transformations that reestablished a normal family atmosphere.

During one of these parent/teacher meetings in April 1980, we discovered, much to our delight, that the children had started conveying events that happened at home and at school. We knew, then, that the children had begun to take on their full stature as speaking subjects and were coming into their own as speaking individuals. In this respect, the purpose of working with the children's parents was to help them recognize their child's verbal abilities by giving them the opportunity to truly communicate with their child through signed French.

We also invited the parents to visit the class. Often it was quite a revelation for them to see their child so interested in speech and able to pay such close attention.

Conclusion: In the Joy of Self-Discovery, the Children Learned to Speak by Playing

Through storytelling, we were able to transport the children back to times past and times never had in their acquisition of language. Only by bringing the children back in time could we offer them the opportunity to experience all the necessary stages in speech acquisition. As they made this journey, the breaches in their relationships began to heal. We saw their faces come alive as their eyes reconnected with those around them — this is what made them once again beautiful and expressive.

With the reestablishment of eye-contact, the children entered into the well-being that envelops stories told for the pleasure of the exchange and the pleasure of *being together*, sharing common feelings and emotions.

Eye-contact also made it possible for us *to anticipate the children's speech*. Stimulated by the speech we offered them *as a gift*, they engaged in a variety of activities to which we then simply responded, respecting that marvelous pedagogy by which mothers draw their children into preverbal dialogue before engaging them in verbal conversation.

Only in Sign Language was such a natural approach to speech in deaf children possible. But since we offered the children vocal speech in parallel with Sign Language, they attributed the same richness to both. The children's ability to acquire visual speech without limitation seemed to compensate for the gaps they inevitably encountered in visually perceiving vocal speech that is meant be heard. Because the children had experienced the fullness of speech in a language thoroughly accessible to them, they were better able to acquire vocal speech. They could not experience all of its characteristics, but they did understand its *uses*.

In a quasi-experimental manner, we were able to see the truth of Diatkine's contention that 'children learn to speak by playing with words' (Diatkine, 1976: 600). Well before using speech to 'say' things, the children *played* with words — visual and vocal alike. They lived out what linguists too often forget: that speech is not so much a *vehicle for content*, as a *connecting process*. As dialogue was reestablished, the children first used speech to play, to connect and to identify with their teachers; only later did they use it to transmit content.

In the following chapter we will broadly examine the stages the children collectively passed through as they entered into speech.

Notes to Chapter 6

1. As in all deaf schools, Sign Language was not recognized or used in this one.
2. Collège d'Etudes Techniques (a technical secondary school).
3. Due to the attention the bilingual class has attracted because of its novelty, we have changed the children's names and omitted any particulars on their backgrounds.
4. Emphasis added.

7 Stages the Children Went Through as They Entered into Speech: September 1979–February 1981

The children were all quite old and still without verbal communication when they enrolled in the class. But within this bilingual setting their extra verbal and verbal interaction developed by leaps and bounds. Here we trace the stages we were able to observe in their development.

But first I would like to express my gratitude to Marie-Thérèse Abbou. Without her collaboration, I could not have understood and interpreted all that the children expressed in Sign.

The Children Rediscover the Pleasure of Eye-Contact and Learn to Synchronize Eye-gaze with Speech

In the dialogue that developed between us through storytelling, the children regained an appetite for establishing eye-contact for the purpose of interaction and communication. But this did not happen overnight. Dialogue gradually revived their visual attention, but at first it remained extremely furtive. For instance, one of the children would look at us when he became interested in the story being told, but as soon as our eyes met he would turn away, gripped by an instinctive urge to avoid others' eyes. Such evasive visual habits gradually diminished and the children would maintain eye-contact for the duration of an utterance.

Once the children had again entered into extra-verbal dialogue and redis-covered the joy of watching someone, they began to understand the role of *eye gaze* in verbal communication. There couldn't have been a better way to help the children make this connection than by immersing them in Sign Language. Sign

173

Language offers deaf children the freedom to watch someone without feeling accosted. They can guardedly catch bits and pieces of what someone is saying to them by looking out of the corners of their eyes or by sneaking furtive glances. This is the same luxury that hearing children enjoy in vocal language: their own desire and willingness dictates what they will and won't listen to out of the flow of words offered them. Even before hearing infants' ears are fully open and attentive to sounds, they pick up something of the verbal activity around them. From time to time a sound will pique their interest and cause them to listen for a little while. But it is their decision whether or not to pay attention with their ears.

Sign Language affords deaf children this same freedom. It is their decision whether or not to pay attention with their eyes to what is said to them.

Because we respected the children's freedom to take only what they wanted of what we offered them, they gradually did become interested in what we had to offer and their eyes followed our storytelling with increasing regularity.

Through Sign Language — the one language that deaf children can fully comprehend and thus receive as a gift — the children moved toward becoming *actively attentive to speech*. Once they discovered the pleasure of watching visual speech, they gradually became interested in watching vocal speech as well, difficult as it was to perceive.

What better preparation for vocal speechreading than to learn a language based on sight? Comfortable and natural communication in Sign Language develops deaf children's visual attention and thus enables them to take an interest in vocal language, which requires sustained and exacting visual attention — the moment concentration lapses and the eyes wander, the thread of speech is lost. In fact, in various discourse situations, even sustained visual attention cannot begin to guarantee comprehension of speech intended to be heard.

Once the children regained their ability to establish and maintain eye-contact with someone speaking to them individually, they then took an interest in what was said to the class as a whole. At first their attention span was very short, but as time went on, it progressively grew longer. Not until early Winter 1980–81 were the children able to repeat a story in unison in Sign Language. They were later able to do this in vocal language as well, though not with the same confidence or consistency.

Besides learning to look at their interlocutor, the children also learned to coordinate their own eye-gaze with verbal expression. That is, they learned to speak and visually register the effect of their speech on their interlocutor at the same time. As Schaffer *et al.* (1977: 322) point out, this kind of integration is what 'gives speech its obviously other-directed character'. It usually develops in children between the ages of one and two years unless particular problems arise.

Though much older, our students were just becoming aware of speech and thus hadn't yet learned to coordinate their eye-gaze and verbalizations. When they first began to express themselves verbally, they often would not look at their interlocutor. For instance, one of the children always looked at the ceiling or the floor when he talked to us in Sign. Whenever we asked him to look at us as he talked, he would stop speaking and refuse to continue. The request probably brought back memories of past experiences when he was aggressed visually. But little by little he began to respond. Instead of blocking us out he would look at us and smile, then start his utterance again while looking into our eyes. As time went on, his eye/speech coordination became increasingly refined.

Such were the hurdles the children had to clear in order to regain visual attention.

Incidentally, when visitors began visiting the class in the Winter of 1979–80, they always went away struck by the students' concentration — these were children who had barely been capable of paying attention at all! Just like any group of children enraptured in an activity, their faces were calm and absorbed. In fact some of the children demonstrated remarkable visual attentiveness. Once, Agnès was off to my side as I spoke to another student, yet she was still able recognize an often used expression on my lips. When the child I was speaking to did not understand, she interpreted the expression for him into Sign Language. Granted, Agnès had the advantage of being our youngest student and the only one to have experienced speech in Sign Language by the age of four. Sabine, on the other hand, was already six years old when she joined the class; she had lost all eye-contact and didn't speak at all. Yet by the Fall of 1980-81, she always demanded everyone's full attention before telling about her weekend. If anyone looked away she would immediately stop her story — she recognized how important eye-contact was to verbal communication.

We must emphasize that deaf children cannot enter into speech at all unless they are capable of paying visual attention. For them, all speech is visual — be it in Sign Language or vocal language. Furthermore, all linguistic communication is based on the way we look at each other as we speak — regardless of whether we are speaking gesturally or vocally. Desmond Morris has shown that eye-gaze is an important part of human interaction and varies greatly in terms of direction and intensity. Such behavior is uniquely human. It is not found in other primates who 'do not stand hour after hour in a face to face relationship, talking to one another. It is, in fact, the evolution of speech that has made eye contact such a significant and useful human signalling device' (Morris, 1977: 75).

Only once the children rediscovered the fundamental role that eyes play in human communication were they able to enter into speech. As their eyes filled with curiosity and attentiveness, their faces filled with beauty.

The Children Acquire Speech to Play with It

As soon as the children became visually attentive, they started picking up words during storytelling. First they acquired clearly 'translucent' units in Sign Language, which they enjoyed reproducing for their physical qualities. But they soon found this same pleasure in repeating vocal words during storytelling in vocal language. These repetitions became the basis for all sorts of verbal interplay.

Playing with words to manipulate them

Since the children played with signifiers in both languages, we will make observations about their playful activities in each.

Manipulating Sign Language

The children's own repetition errors were often what brought them to play with signifiers. Sometimes these errors arose from *articulation difficulties*. The children usually managed to use the correct placement, movement and orientation of a sign, but sometimes had trouble forming the correct handshape. Lacking manual dexterity, they had troubles extending their fingers or holding them in. (Marina McIntire (1977) observed these same difficulties in her research on the acquisition of American Sign Language.) Rémi, for instance, could not make the 'J' handshape (cf. manual alphabet, page 96) because he could not extend his thumb and little finger while holding down his other fingers. Consequently, he had problems forming any sign made with this handshape (e.g. PETIT, JOUER, JAUNE). He also could not hold his thumb in against the side of his palm to form the 'B' or 'G' handshapes. Whenever he signed a word made with one of these handshapes (e.g. BLEU, BATEAU, GARÇON, ROUGE, FILLE), his thumb stuck out instead of lying against the palm. But with support from the deaf teacher, who molded the children's hands into the correct shape, these difficulties disappeared within a few months. By March 1980, we observed that Rémi — the child most prone to this type of problem — only made handshape errors from time to time. In October 1980, he even took it upon himself to correct a hearing adult who signed BLEU with her thumb sticking out — the very same mistake he had systematically made a year earlier.

Patrick, on the other hand, had an articulation problem connected with muscle tone. His signs were always extremely tense. But little by little he learned to control his movements and to soften his articulation. He would sometimes even repeat a sign over and over to experiment with different degrees of tension.

Sometimes the children's errors arose not from any articulatory problem, but from *difficulties in phonological analysis*; that is, they would confuse two very similar signs, such as *minimal sign pairs*, which differ only in a single parameter. Listed below is an example of each type of confusion we observed:

OU /	JOUER	Confusion between two signs that are identical
(or)	(play)	*except in handshape.*
MONSIEUR /	IL Y A	Confusion between two signs that are identical
(Mister)	(there is/are)	*except in placement.*
PRETER /	POUSSIERE	Confusion between two signs that are identical
(loan)	(dust)	*except in movement.*
MARDI /	SAMEDI	Confusion between two signs that are identical
(Tuesday)	(Saturday)	*except in orientation.*
MAL /	CONTENT	Confusion between two signs that are identical
(badly, hurt)	(happy)	*except in facial expression.*

In addition to confusing minimal sign pairs, the children also confused signs having two characteristics in common. The signs most frequently confused were those with identical placement and handshape: AIDER (help) and CAMPAGNE (countryside), MOURIR (die) and REPONDRE (answer), etc.

The deaf teacher would provide the children with a proper verbal model, bringing their attention to the phonological differences they had not noticed. Learning from their own errors and the corrections, the children became attentive to signifiers and began to play with them. They started making observations about various similarities and differences between signs. On 19th November 1980, for example, we were telling that week's story about a dog that kept watch over sheep. This time Charles picked up the new sign GARDER (keep watch), repeated it to himself, and then told the deaf teacher that this sign resembled the sign POUSSIERE (dust) — introduced three weeks earlier in a story that Charles had really liked about little houses of different colors. GARDER and POUSSIERE in fact form a minimal pair, differing only in movement.

Having developed this metalinguistic perspective on sign formation, the children began asking for clarifications. On 20th November 1980, for instance, we presented a new story about a heroine named Hélène. Sabine asked the deaf teacher if the name-sign HELENE was made by repeating it two or three times. The sign does involve repeating a movement — Sabine simply had not caught how many times.

The children also became interested in each other's signing and began to correct each other. This game started in November 1979 with the children immediately imitating the deaf teacher whenever she corrected a student's sign. One of the children would get up and show the others how well he or she could make the sign by imitating exactly what the teacher did. This game spontaneously led the children to begin correcting each other. In the Fall of 1980, for instance, Linda took great delight in correcting Sabine when she signed NEIGE (snow) with the wrong handshape.

Sometimes the children even delved into full-blown phonological analyses. When Charles asked if the signs SAINT-JACQUES and DEMAIN (tomorrow) were the same, Agnès answered by showing him the difference and explaining in Sign Language that if one is not careful DEMAIN can be mistaken for SAINT-JACQUES, L'ECOLE (the Saint Jacques school). These two signs, identical in handshape and placement, were among those the children easily confused. On another occasion, it was Charles who corrected Agnès when she said MORT (dead) instead of RENTRER (return), confusing these very similar signs. He showed her the difference and told her vocally, 'Pas "mort"'.

When the children knew a synonym for a sign used by the teacher, they would offer it spontaneously. For example, Linda proudly showed that she knew another sign for MORT. And Agnès did likewise with GRONDER (scold).

The children were very active metalingually and could even indicate when they didn't understand a new sign. For instance, when some deaf friends from the South of France came to visit the class and used a different sign for ROSE (pink), the children asked them for an explanation. The children engaged in similar activities at home, correcting their parents if they formed a sign incorrectly, and showing them new signs they had learned.

One observation in particular illustrates just how quickly and intensely the children took an interest in signifiers: In April 1980 Sabine commented that her deaf teacher had made a mistake when telling a story on TV. The teacher had formed the sign OURS (bear) with a three-finger instead of a five-finger claw handshape. This child, remember, had joined the class the previous September with utterly blank eyes and enormous attention problems.

The above-described manipulations always involved isolated words. Yet the children also played with whole sentences as they recited stories in unison and engaged in reading activities. They loved to repeat sentences that were written on the board and tried to memorize them for the mere pleasure of being able to produce them again. This was not serious speech for 'saying' something; it was speech for play.

Once the children accomplished an activity in Sign Language there was always a slight time lag before they could do it in vocal language. Yet when it came to metalinguistic activities, this time lag was nearly imperceptible.

Manipulating Vocal Language

Once the children knew a story in Sign Language, they enjoyed picking up vocal words from the vocal language narrative. Just for fun they would repeat those words whose meaning and lip pattern were clear. As we know, facial expressions play an important role in Sign Language, serving phonological and syntactic functions as well as expressive ones. Yet facial expressions also come into play in vocal language as they accompany the lip movements of speech. In storytelling, these facial expressions often become more pronounced to reflect the emotion of the situation. Vocal words thus become 'translucent' like signed words. The relationship between their form and their content becomes apparent when the content is known. Take, for example, the French word *tigre*. In one story, there is a part where 'the tiger is going to eat the little boy'. In this context, our articulation of the word *tigre* [pronounced tee-gre] could evoke the animal — the face and lip movements of the first phonemes [ti] suggesting the tiger's feline characteristics, and the last phonemes [gr] suggesting its roar. Yet when this same word is spoken in a completely neutral speech situation, it is barely even visible on the lips.

The translucency of emphatically produced vocal words enabled the children to recognize key words in the story. Let it be clear that *emphasizing* words did not mean *deforming* them — they were always pronounced naturally without altering the normal lip pattern. Just as in all child-directed speech, emphasis was achieved simply by saying words more slowly and accompanying them with amplified facial expression.

Once the children began recognizing vocal words, they soon made attempts to produce them. Even though they didn't always use their voice, they would reproduce the lip patterns of the words they recognized. Happy to see these efforts, the hearing teacher would give the children encouraging feedback, showing that she understood what they were trying to say. In fact, she was often amazed at what the children were able to do, and made no effort to hide her admiration. The children eagerly attempted to produce vocal words, for they were happy to be understood and proud of the positive reflection they received of themselves.

As of Winter 1979–80 the children were able to repeat in unison a story told in vocal language. These repetitions were at first rather broken and limited to lexical words. Grammatical words, which are often monosyllabic and unstressed, were virtually impossible for the children to perceive visually in the short sentences they repeated after us. In order to maintain all the natural intonations of speech, we never stressed anything that should not be stressed. Right from the start, the children were taught natural sentence rhythm, which would greatly enhance the intelligibility of their vocal speech in the future.

At the end of Spring 1980, we witnessed a new behavior in the children. Right in the middle of storytelling one of them would get up, stop everything, and with obvious pleasure vocally articulate for everyone a particular word he or she had been practicing during the story. If not convinced that all the other children had been watching, the child would go around and say the word right in front of each person — including the deaf teacher. Both teachers would applaud and the storytelling would resume. Interestingly, the children always concentrated for a brief moment before vocally producing a word for the others — a clear indication that they were *actively acquiring vocal speech.*

Parallel to this development, the children also began translating into Sign Language the vocal words they recognized through speechreading. This behavior developed from the hearing teacher's habit of asking them for the signs that corresponded to the vocal words they repeated. This was to ensure that the children weren't simply 'parroting' her. This kind of translation became an important activity in the Fall of 1981. The children began to emulate each other's eagerness to be the first to translate what the hearing teacher said. In fact in January 1981, their parents informed us that the children had introduced this activity at home: they would say something vocally, playing the part of the hearing teacher, and then ask their parents for a translation in signs. The parents did their very best to understand these early attempts at vocal speech so as not to discourage their child, now confident in his or her verbal abilities — in a vocal modality, no less.

By systematically playing these translation games, the children gained extensive practice in speechreading. We were pleased to see that they began making translation errors because they were confusing words that were very similar, if not identical, on the lips. Such confusion showed that their receptive acquisition of vocal speech had truly taken root. When we told the story about differently colored houses (30th September 1980), we knew that Sabine had speechread *mange* (eat) instead of *blanche* (white) because she signed MANGE to translate the word *blanche* articulated by the teacher. Being very familiar with the word *mange*, Sabine had projected its image on to a word having a very similar lip pattern (simply articulate the two words in front of a mirror to see for yourself). The very same day, Linda mistook *brûle* (burn) for *bleu* (blue), which has an identical lip pattern. This showed how fully she had internalized the visual form of the word *bleu*. Both words, in fact, appear in this story: 'the little pink house burns' and 'the little blue house dances'.

Incidentally, such confusion between words did not usually occur upon the first telling of a story, but later on when the children had become familiar with the content of what was said and could *make hypotheses* about the verbal productions they perceived.

The children were delighted when they realized that they could understand what was said with lips. This was particularly clear in Patrick. The very first time he recognized a word on the lips he was so excited he could hardly contain himself as he translated it into Sign Language. Upon entering the class, Patrick had paid no attention to others' faces and had no idea that the lips could even carry meaning.

The children became so interested in vocal speech that they even began correcting what each other said vocally. When, in the Fall of 1980, Patrick said *neige* without its final consonant, Linda corrected him by showing him the word's proper lip pattern with the final [ʒ]. Such incidents revealed how attentive the children had become to each other, even when it came to vocal speech. Interestingly, Linda had recently corrected another child (Sabine) who had signed NEIGE with the wrong handshape. Able to manipulate Sign Language without obstacle, the children seemed to apply these same activities quite readily to vocal language, even though their abilities were much more limited in this language that they could not fully perceive.

. The children began using their speech therapy sessions as an opportunity to continue and refine their analyses and observations of vocal speech. They eagerly awaited their turn, sometimes even arguing over who got to go next. In these sessions, the children were given the chance to improve what they had attempted during the group lesson. In this context, they gradually became interested in auditory exercises. The bits of sound the children managed to pick up became significant because vocal speech was now meaningful to them. Not uncommonly, the children would interrupt the class upon returning from speech therapy to show the other children and the teachers what they had just learned to say vocally.

One observation in particular illustrates how meaningful vocal speech had become to the children. One week in June 1980, we told a story that the children really enjoyed about an old boat. At that time, Agnès had not yet mastered the phoneme [t] and thus had troubles saying the word *bateau*, which came up again and again throughout the story. Agnès had been working on her [t] for months; all week long she tried extra hard in her individual sessions to articulate this word *bateau*. Finally, on the last day of the week, she succeeded. A deaf friend of the deaf teacher was visiting the class that day. A few moments before the class let out, the two deaf adults began chatting together in animated conversation. The children were spellbound, watching them with hungry eyes. Happy that the children had this opportunity to observe speech not directed at them — something that happened all to rarely — the hearing teacher let them watch and went into an adjoining room to organize some papers. What a surprise when in came Agnès, her cheeks flushed with pride and satisfaction, to offer a perfectly articulated [bato]! Her accomplishment was so important to her that she had got up and left the group of enraptured children to go and inform the hearing teacher of her breakthrough achieved during her individual session with the other speech therapist. This illustrates how keenly interested deaf children can become in vocal speech once they discover the pleasures of verbal communication.

Vocal speech inevitably presents difficulties for children who cannot hear it. Yet the children in our class intently applied themselves to manipulating signifiers in *both languages* — vocal language as well as Sign Language. Playing with signifiers in each language seemed to be their way identifying with the deaf and hearing people around them.

Playing with words to establish identities

We expected the children to enjoy manipulating signs immensely, but were surprised when they also took enormous pleasure in manipulating vocal speech, which they could not even fully perceive. We also expected the children to prefer working with the deaf teacher over working with the hearing teacher. But this was not the case at all. If the deaf teacher went a bit over time in an activity, one of the children would always let her know that her 'turn' was up by signing MAINTENANT, DANIELLE PARLE (now, Danielle speak). Since all our activities were done first in one language and then in the other, this meant 'now we want to work in vocal language'. Some days, when the time came to repeat a story, the children would say that it was tiring to talk with their hands and that they preferred to speak with their mouths. We noticed on occasion that some of the children were now more attentive when the story was being told by the hearing teacher than by the deaf teacher — a real switch from when they were just beginning to speak (cf. page 173). This tended to happen toward the end of the week when the children were very familiar with a story in Sign Language and thus had no trouble following it on the lips of a hearing person.

In our estimation, the children's attraction to vocal language stemmed from their need to identify with their hearing teacher since she resembled their parents and other family members and acquaintances. Yet the children could not have *established identities through vocal language* had they not first discovered the various functions of speech *through Sign Language*. It is because they had received a verbal model offered by a deaf person that they came to exist as full speaking subjects and to understand that *to speak is to find one's identity*. By identifying with their deaf teacher, the children knew they were deaf. They were able to situate themselves *vis-à-vis* their parents and to understand the ways in which they were different. They thus recognized vocal speech as a prime means of satisfying their need to identify with their parents.

Only *bilingual education* offers deaf children the adult reference models they need to discover themselves and to identify with people from the hearing and deaf worlds to which they belong. Speech seems to play a leading role in the subtle dialectic by which children develop their various identifications. This would explain why the children in our class were so earnest in learning to speak vocally.

The children's speech-based identifications became apparent in many different ways. For instance, when Charles distributed folders to the other children during an activity with the deaf teacher, he would call out their names in Sign Language by using their name-signs. But when he distributed the folders during an activity with the hearing teacher, he would call out the children's names vocally, and they would watch his lips to catch their name. The children thus showed great flexibility in switching from one language to another depending on the speech situation.

Whenever the children met someone new, they always wanted to know immediately whether the person was deaf or hearing. They had a clear sense of the two worlds in which they would always live, and seemed to have reached this awareness primarily through speech. By manipulating speech in many different ways, the children also quickly came to understand that speech is a way to make contact with others.

Playing with words to make contact

During this period of speech acquisition through playing with signifiers, we observed the following phenomenon: The children sought to connect with us by producing 'discourse' strangely similar to speech in Sign Language, but which incorporated only two or three recognizable signs. With obvious pleasure, the children would 'talk' to us using all sorts of hand movements and facial expressions that resembled Sign Language. In fact, the hearing teacher had the impression that the children were speaking in Sign Language with such dexterity that she couldn't follow what they were saying. But the deaf teacher couldn't make head or tail of it either, though it was strangely similar to 'her' language in its beauty and gestural intonation.

Similar situations arise with hearing children when they are just beginning to talk at around age two. Here is one account, related by Christine Leroy (1975):

Some foreign friends remarked on how surprised they were to hear little 18-month-old N. L. speak 'such perfect French'. These friends, who had been living in France for only a few months, were convinced that N. L. was speaking 'standard' language because the intonation patterns and sounds he made were acoustically very similar to what they heard around them, from the mouths of other adults. At the time, N. L. had barely fifteen 'words' that his parents could honestly interpret! (Leroy, 1975: 40)

The child's vocal activity was such that, to a foreign ear, he seemed to be speaking.

Children seem to discover the connecting process involved in speech and use it to satisfy their need for contact before they can effectively 'speak up'. They go on and on in what appears to be verbal activity while actually reproducing nothing more than its most suggestive formal characteristics. In vocal language, children simply make sounds in intonation patterns that resemble those of real discourse; and in gestural language, they perform perfectly imitative gestures and movements.

On 20th March 1980, at a time when Sabine was not yet capable of recounting her weekend as some of the other children could, she delivered a long speech when it came her turn to talk. 'It's beautiful to watch', exclaimed the deaf teacher. 'It looks like a poetic form of Sign Language, yet I can't understand any of it except for a few signs that stand out from the gestural flow'. This observation was strikingly similar to Leroy's account of the 18-month-old who seemed to deliver whole speeches though he had a vocabulary of only fifteen 'words'. Such behavior tended to disappear once the children were able to use speech to transmit information. Yet it did resurface from time to time. We observed one such recurrence in Linda on 29th September 1980. Although she had finished describing her weekend, she felt that her story had been too short. So she continued on in a gestural imitation of Sign Language in order to keep the deaf teacher's attention and to keep her turn.

In sum, playing with words certainly did seem to lead to speech used to 'say' something, to transmit content.

The Children Acquire Speech to Transmit Content

Once the children acquired words by playing with their signifiers as described above, they began to 'speak up' to say things and to express themselves. At first, language had been *an object of knowledge* in the extra-verbal and verbal communication surrounding storytelling. But it then became *a means of expressing and telling about oneself*. The two children who joined the class in September 1979 without any verbal communication, began spontaneously expressing themselves by the end of the first quarter. As she entered the class-room on 7th December 1979, Sabine said to us in Sign 'SABINE EST TOMBEE VOITURE' (Sabine fell car), to say that she had fallen down in the street. Even without knowing the sign RUE (street), she had still made herself understood; the deaf teacher was able to offer her appropriate feedback on what she had meant to say. During that same period, Rémi always asked the deaf teacher to repeat the story of Father Christmas. In turn, he would make a few short statements in Sign Language regarding Father Christmas: 'PERE NOEL ENTRE DANS LA MAISON' (Father Christmas enters the house)...'REMI DORT' (Rémi is sleeping). During the Winter of 1980, such *spontaneous verbalizations* became increasingly frequent. Interestingly, the signs the children used to express themselves were those they had seen over and over again in our storytelling (see page 166).

During storytelling, the children no longer merely anticipated isolated signs or short statements, but began telling the story themselves. On 21st February 1980, during a story about a lost kitten, Agnès jumped in signing 'PAPA ACHETE LE PANIER' (Daddy buys the basket)... 'IL ARRIVE A LA MAISON' (he arrives home). Likewise, on 28th February Sabine interrupted a story about a little red hen to say in Sign: 'ELLE FAIT UN GATEAU' (she makes a cake), 'QUI M'AIDE?' (who will help me?). And on 11th March during a story about a baby bear too young to do things by himself, Rémi took the lead, signing 'PAPA OURS S'HABILLE' (Papa bear gets dressed), 'IL VIENT AVEC LUI' (he comes with him [with the baby bear]), 'IL PART AU MARCHE' (he goes to market). In all of these instances, the children were anticipat-ing what would happen next. In their early storytelling, the children did not make original statements but recounted the events of a story as it had been told to them. At the time, only Charles developed stories of his own by making up an original ending or adding details here and there. For example, on 24th January 1980, we told a story in which the hero drops a coin into a river. Charles embellished this event saying, 'LA PIECE TOME SUR LE POISSON QUI TOURNE DANS L'EAU' (the coin hits the fish that is swimming around in the water). As time went on, the other children also began telling their own versions of stories. On 19th November 1980, for instance, we told a story about a worthless dog who did not know how to keep watch over sheep and ended up making them scatter. Agnès added in a detail, explaining that the wolf was going to eat them...just as he had tried to eat the baby goats. She then launched into a story about the baby goats and how the mama-goat came to save them just as the wolf was about to eat them. We had told the children this story a year earlier, during the week of 6th November 1979! This showed how important storytelling was to the children's imagination and how instrumental these stories were in helping them to express themselves in sto-ries of their own creation. In fact, when the children started contributing to sto-ries, their personal embellishments almost always explicitly referred to some story they had already been told, as did Agnès' in the above example.

Once the children were able to produce these little story-based narratives, they also became capable of talking about what they did at home. This started after the Easter vacation, 1980. At that time, the quality of these accounts varied enormously from one child to the next. Agnès and Charles expressed themselves very clearly, and were able to let everyone know what they had done over the vacation: Agnès had gone to the mountains with her friend Linda, and Charles had gone to see his grandmother who had some geese. Sabine and Rémi were much more difficult to understand. In Sabine's account, there were a few recognizable sentences such as 'LA NUIT, MOI JE DORS DANS LA VOITURE' (At night, I sleep in the car), but the rest was a gestural imitation of Sign Language. Sabine clearly enjoyed telling about herself and didn't want to relinquish her turn for lack of linguistic ability. Rémi took a different approach. He expressed himself with a few isolated signs enveloped in a whole production of blackboard drawings and facial expressions. For all their desire to make themselves understood, these two children's explanations were difficult to follow. This showed that the use of language truly was a 'miracle of communication' (Perron-Borelli, 1976: 690) that had not yet happened for Sabine and Rémi. But gradually it did: on 21st April 1980 Rémi (absent the day before) arrived at school saying that his grandmother had been sick (it was she who brought him to school) and that he had played with cars in his room.

As time went on the children's stories became much clearer and true linguistic communication developed between us. Once the children became more comfortable telling their stories, we began seeing signs of metalinguistic activity in the way they constructed their utterances. In telling about her weekend on 22st September 1980, Agnès padded her statements with 'A CAUSE DE' (on account of, owing to) — an expression she had recently learned. Interestingly, she also paused for a moment before uttering each statement, as though to organize her sentences. She also backtracked. She would begin speaking, then stop and begin again in a different way. A week later, on 29th September we observed similar behavior in Charles. Intent on fully appropriating the expression 'PARCE QUE' (because), he used it in each and every one of his statements. And on 17th November Linda played with 'POUR' (for, in order to) in a similar way, using it in every utterance whether it was appropriate or not. During this same period, Sabine showed signs of metalingual activity using the Sign Language device of indicating a point in space as an anaphoric marker. She employed this technique to the point of redundancy. This is similar to when hearing children repeat a subject in vocal language, saying, for instance, 'Mommy, *she* bought me an ice cream'. Sabine's linguistic behavior showed that she was actively appropriating this particular Sign Language device for establishing pronouns.

In short, the children were visibly developing a series of syntactic 'schemata' by feeling their way and experimenting. As Lentin says of all children learning to speak, 'They make hypotheses, experiment with them, and make progress, just like a researcher' (Lentin, 1973: 57). This was certainly true of each of the children in our class.

As they told their stories, they paid astonishingly close attention to each other. There were even times when the more advanced students would translate for the teachers what another child was trying to tell them. The children were all eager to express themselves, but they waited their turn to speak and would not cut off another child's story. For instance, one day when Linda obviously had nothing more to say but was dragging out her story for her own pleasure, Agnès said to her, 'C'EST LONG!', 'ENCORE LONGTEMPS?' 'NOUS, ON ATTEND, ON ATTEND...' (It's long! Much longer? Us, we're waiting, we're waiting).

Once the children were able to tell stories to an adult, they began *to converse among themselves.* Here is one such exchange — about a lost pen — that took place between Linda and Charles on 22nd September 1980:

L: OU? CE MATIN, AUTOUR DU COU, LE STYLO.
Where? This morning around the neck, the pen.

C: AH OUI! A LA CANTINE J'AI OUBLIE.
Oh yes! At lunch I forgot.

(Verbal units expressed in proper Sign Language order.)

L: DEMAIN, TU CHERCHES.
Tomorrow, you search.

(Proper use of indexing — a Sign Language grammatical device.)

C: DEMAIN, JE CHERCHE A LA CANTINE, MONSIEUR BARBU.
Tomorrow, I search at lunch, bearded man.

On 28th November Sabine and Charles had this conversation about the weather:

S: IL FAIT BEAU TEMPS.
The weather is nice.

C: NON.
No.

S: SI! LE SOLEIL EST PARTI.
Yes! The sun is gone.

(Statement in Signed French, with signs corresponding to the words of the French sentence. In French Sign Language one would say, 'LE SOLEIL A DISPARU' ('The sun has disappeared'.))

One Sunday in November 1980 all the children were invited to Linda's house for her birthday party. Here is an excerpt from their interaction as they told about it in class:

Sabine: LINDA ET PATRICK ONT FAIT DU VELO. PATRICK M'A DONNE UN COUP DE PIED.
Linda and Patrick rode bikes. Patrick kicked me.

(Sabine clearly indicates the agent and the object of the verb in Sign Language by the direction of her movement in signing 'DONNER'.)

AGNES RIEN, PAS DE VELO. MAQUILLEE.
Agnès nothing, no bike. Make-up on.

(Agnès speaks up)

Agnès: POUR ETRE BELLE.
To be pretty.

(Sabine concedes and continues her story,
which will again be interrupted by Agnès.)

Sabine: MOI, J'ETAIS SALE.
Me, I was dirty.

Agnes: PARCE QU'ELLE EST TOMBEE CONTRE LE SAPIN
Because she fell against the pine tree.

(Another statement in Signed French — the words are in French word order. In Sign Language one would say, 'LE SAPIN, ELLE EST TOMBEE CONTRE' (The pine tree, she fell against).)

(Sabine disagrees with Agnès' explanation)

Sabine: NON! C'EST PATRICK QUI M'A DONNE UN COUP DE PIED.
No! Patrick kicked me.

(Linda gets impatient.)

Linda: ALLEZ! CONTINUEZ A RACONTER!
Come on, get on with the story!

This example shows how well the children could say exactly what they meant and carry on a true linguistic exchange among themselves.

Once the children were able to converse with each other in this way, they found they could satisfy their need for interaction with each other as partners. They then became more independent. This was good for their psychological development and also relieved their teachers from feeling monopolized.

It must be emphasized, however, that the children could not have begun to speak to each other had they not each experienced linguistic interaction with adults. Children do not learn to speak from each other unless they have enjoyed privileged interaction with adult partners who offer them a *verbal model* adapted to their linguistic development.

In January 1981, we were pleasantly surprised by the effectiveness of our verbal exchanges with the children. They were now able to respond clearly and easily. Two examples illustrate the atmosphere of verbal communication that had developed. One day Sabine fingerspelled a word. Surprised that she knew how, the hearing teacher asked her, 'QUI T'A APPRIS A' (Who taught you that?). Sabine's answer was very specific — she gave the name of the deaf person who visited her family once a week. The dialogue was quick, clear and to the point, and had provided the desired explanation. On another occasion, the deaf teacher did a Charlie Chaplin imitation as she talked to Rémi about the actor. Rémi responded saying, 'AH OUI!, JE CONNAIS, J'AI VU A LA TELEVISION' (Oh yeah! I know, I saw on television). He then did an imitation of Charlie Chaplin, too. Here again, the exchange was clear. Our communication with the children thus became increasingly satisfying while our frustrations diminished relative to their capacity for interaction.

In sum, the children became adept at translating their thoughts into words. When they returned to school from the Christmas vacation in January 1981, they were all able to clearly recount what they had done and to describe in great detail the presents they had received.

About this time, the children learned to say 'JE N'AI PAS COMPRIS' (I didn't understand) when they were unable to follow our speech, and 'JE NE SAIS PAS' (I don't know) when they did not know the answer to a question. The children's ability to clearly distinguish between code-related and content-related obstacles to an exchange showed how comfortable they had become with situating themselves in verbal interactions. The distinction also attested to the children's command of interrelated *metalinguistic* and *referential* activities.

For all their verbal interactions, the children resorted primarily to signing. By February 1981, Charles and Agnès almost always accompanied their signing with fairly intelligible vocal speech, but the other children did so only with a few of their signs. The words they produced in this dual vocal-gestural mode were those they had most fully appropriated from the stories we told: *non* (no), *après* (after), *beaucoup* (a lot, many), *peut pas* (can't), *cherche* (look for), *perdu* (lost), *sale* (dirty), *beau* (beautiful), *papa* (daddy), *maman* (mommy), *lapin* (rabbit), the names of colors, etc. Incidentally, both Charles and Agnès had also gone through a stage when they vocalized words with only a few signs. In fact they still made signs without their vocal equivalent if they did not know what it was. Agnès, for example, never said anything vocally when she signed FER A REPASSER (iron) because she didn't know how.

Interestingly, the children used both a gestural and vocal modality simulta-neously whenever they knew the vocal equivalents to their signs. This was a *regular behavior*. The children seemed to enjoy making such connections when-ever they could.

As the children appropriated Sign Language word order and the techniques of repetition, localization and directionality, their 'simultaneously signed and vocalized' utterances began to conform to Sign Language syntax. Sometimes, however, these bimodal utterances followed vocal language syntax, as seen in the two instances of Signed French in the child-to-child conversations tran-scribed above. The children could thus be observed acquiring the syntax of both languages.

As the following examples clearly show, the children were able to distin-guish the two languages even though they used the same bimodal (gestural/vocal) means of expression for both. In a discussion about Helen Keller on 21st November 1980, Sabine said 'PEUT PAS PARLER' (can't speak) to the hearing teacher and then turned and said 'PARLER PEUT PAS' (speak can't) to the deaf teacher. In other words, she addressed each teacher in her own language, respecting the different treatment of negatives in each of the two languages. In this case, Sabine was *repeating statements* that each of the teachers had formu-lated over and over again as they told the story of Helen Keller. But she made a similar distinction in her own *spontaneous statements*. For instance she would say 'MECHANT PAS' (mean not) according to Sign Language syntax or 'PAS MECHANT' (not mean), following vocal language syntax depending on whom she was talking to.

Similarly, Agnès employed the syntactic construction proper to each lan-guage when expressing the iterative aspect in her spontaneous statements. In recounting her February vacation, she used the repetitive Sign Language con-struction 'JE SORS, JE SORS, JE SORS' (I go out, I go out, I go out) to explain that she went out all the time because the weather was so nice. Yet just a few days earlier she had said, 'JE SORS TOUJOURS' (I always go out) to express the same idea. Here she used vocal language syntax, expressing the iterative aspect in the form of an adverb. The term 'always' does exist in Sign Language, but does not seem to be used as an iterative marker.

Thus, the children's 'simultaneously signed and vocalized' utterances — which at the outset followed a grammar all of their own, as do the statements of all children just learning to speak — gradually conformed to either Sign Language syntax or vocal language syntax. One may see children speaking with their hands, but this does not necessarily mean that they are speaking in Sign Language.

Figure 7.1 helps define these notions of *bimodality* and *bilingualism*:

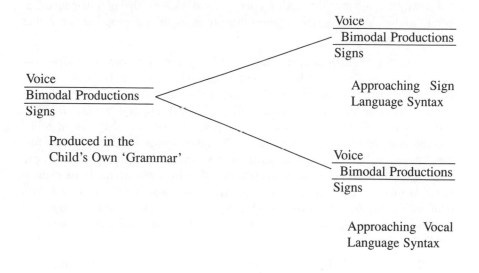

FIGURE 7.1

Through expressing themselves bimodally, the children entered into both languages we offered them. As deaf children, however, they appropriated the syntactic structures of Sign Language more quickly than those of vocal language. Sign Language matches deaf children's abilities and enables them to discover grammatical notions and relationships because, in this language, they are expressed in a fully accessible visual modality. Deaf children can then better comprehend these same notions in a vocal language whose formal characteristics they are far from being able to grasp. Once familiar with grammatical relationships in a language that comes to them naturally, deaf children are able to infer these same relationships in vocal language through mental guesswork and what little they can perceive. This is another reason why true bilingual education is so essential for deaf children. Signed French may vastly improve their ability to interact linguistically, but it does not allow them to begin experimenting with syntax in any coherent way. The syntax of a *temporally* organized language, based on linear acoustical constructions, will necessarily differ significantly from the syntax of a *spatially* organized language based on signs. Consequently, signs produced in vocal language word order lose all the inflectional variations based on the logic of spatially-defined syntax. Signed French is indispensable in family communication between *hearing* parents and a *deaf* child; yet along with Signed French, deaf children must be exposed to Sign Language so they can coherently acquire the grammatical concepts and relationships of a language that comes to them naturally. This enables them to more fully appropriate the syntax of vocal language.

Once the children started using Sign Language and vocal language syntax, they seemed better able to respect the mode in which language is normally expressed. Starting in late February 1981, Agnès began using only her voice when uttering statements that followed vocal language syntax. By venturing to express herself without the support of gestures, she seemed to be gaining confidence in her vocalizations. In other words Agnès, who was furthest along in her language acquisition, had truly begun to speak in *vocal language* not only in terms of syntax, but also in terms of mode of expression. At this point in her development, Agnès was also able to converse with deaf adults in *Sign Language* respecting both its syntax and its mode of expression by using only signs. In sum, Agnès had undeniably begun to speak *two languages*.

By Spring 1980, it was clear that the children should start attending a full day of school in September. Not only had their capacity for paying attention returned to normal, but they were thirsting for knowledge. The two hours we spent with the children each day was no longer enough. In addition to learning speech in a bilingual setting, they also needed to begin their formal education.

We began searching for a school that would agree to enroll the children in regular morning classes and allow us to take them for the afternoon to continue working on verbal communication.

This arrangement allowed the children to experience being integrated into an ordinary school. In the following sections we discuss various aspects of that experience.

September 1980: The Children Integrate into the Life of a School for Hearing Children

In September 1980, a school practicing 'active' teaching methods agreed to accept the children according to the proposed arrangement. Four of them were integrated into the second grade class and the other two, Agnès and Rémi, were placed in first grade.[1] (Agnès wasn't yet old enough for 2nd grade, and at the time Rémi didn't quite have the mental balance that the constraints and pace of 2nd grade would require.)

Even though the children were intellectually capable of following the activities of their respective classes, their profound deafness meant they would completely miss all instructions and information given in the usual verbal mode. We knew that we would have to provide the children with a Sign Language interpreter in order for them to benefit fully from the class time they spent in a hearing environment. Integrating the children into hearing classes was, in fact, inconceivable without an interpreter. Only with an interpreter would they be truly accepted — respected for their difference and acknowledged in their identity.

A speech therapist having a solid command of Sign Language and working toward an interpreting degree served as the children's interpreter, dividing her time between the two classes. It was important that the interpreter had been trained as a speech therapist — she was addressing young children just learning to speak and just starting school.

How the children were perceived at school

With their language recognized through the presence of an interpreter, the children were perceived more as foreigners who spoke a different language than as handicapped children. This attitude was apparent in many of the hearing children's comments. When the interpreter translated a comment that Charles' teacher made to him about his birthday cake, a hearing child remarked to the student sitting next to him, 'You see, she's translating for him and now he will understand...'. For these young hearing students deafness did not mean being unable to speak and understand, it meant needing to speak differently. For them, deaf children were — like them — *children who talked*. The hearing children identified with them and accepted them as equals, even in terms of speech. For instance, when a hearing child saw Charles and Linda talking to each other in signs, he asked the interpreter to translate for him what they were saying.

The interpreter's main function in the classroom was to translate what the teacher said to the class as a whole as well as all the asides between an individual student and the teacher. This enabled the deaf children to understand what was happening. When the children were free to talk with each other in between activities or during relaxed activity times, the interpreter was also called upon by deaf and hearing children alike to assist them in communicating with each other. For instance at one point a hearing child asked the interpreter how to say 'May I borrow your eraser?' so that he could go and ask one of the deaf children.

As time went on the hearing children acquired quite a vocabulary of signs, and real communication, including verbal communication, developed between them and the deaf students. Children, of course, always manage to communicate with each other, even if only at a motor or body level. But the interpreter's presence seemed to encourage the children to *use speech* to achieve their exchanges. While the hearing children acquired signs, the deaf children tried their hardest to speak vocally when they conversed with other children. While they were recognized as having their own language, they also wanted very much to speak like their hearing friends.

Such an atmosphere of real interaction among children seems to be a key factor in how well a deaf person will integrate into hearing society as he or she grows older. If deaf people shared life and friendship with their hearing peers in early childhood, they wouldn't feel inferior to them in adulthood. As it is, the deaf invariably say they experience feelings of inferiority *vis-à-vis* hearing people from whom they were separated in school. Those who were integrated into hearing schools never had an interpreter because Sign Language — the one language they could fully perceive — was not acknowledged. 'Integration' as they knew it was nothing more than juxtaposition — a situation in which they were made painfully aware of the chasm separating them from their hearing classmates who had no trouble understanding vocal speech or following class activities. And juxtaposition quickly turns to exclusion.

How Sign Language was perceived at school

After we had been at the school for a few months, a ten-year-old girl approached the deaf teacher and myself as we chatted on the playground, and asked me to translate the following message for the deaf teacher: 'I wouldn't want to be deaf, but I would really like to know how to talk with my hands'. Her words and manner showed a real subtly of feeling and revealed how much Sign Language fascinated her. All the hearing children wanted to learn the basics of this language that seemed to offer unimagined possibilities for communication. Often they would come up to either the deaf or hearing teacher and ask how to say some often-used expression such as 'What's your name?' in Sign Language.

Likewise, the school's regular faculty and staff were eager to attend the weekly Sign Language class we provided after school. They wanted to be able to understand and interact with the deaf children when passing them in the hallway or supervising them in the cafeteria or on the playground. Like the hearing children, they found Sign Language to be both rich and beautiful.

With an interpreter to facilitate classroom communication, and having learned enough Sign Language to communicate somewhat on their own, the two teachers who had the deaf children in their regular classes did not experience any real increase in workload. In fact they noticed that the interpreter's visual speech sometimes helped keep the class calm and attentive.

Parents at the school had nothing against their children attending school with deaf children. In fact, they saw the deaf students as a positive influence. Because of their presence, their hearing children had developed a keen interest in Sign Language and expanded their horizons to another mode of communication. During a parents meeting, they voiced such reactions as, 'Our children are delighted — they know many signs, even sentences... It must be very enriching for them'.

In short, Sign Language — scoffed at in specialized circles — was very well received and even admired in an ordinary school. Such positive attitudes toward Sign Language can't help but positively affect the manner in which deaf children are integrated into hearing schools; when Sign Language is admired, so are those who speak it.

The children's experience in a hearing school could in fact serve as a model for migrant children, who also should be able to attend schools where knowing another language is valued as a real asset. In such an atmosphere, majority-language children are eager to learn the minority language of a classmate who is different from them; and respect develops toward the person whose language is respected. According to the World Center for Information on Bilingual Education,[2] *true integration of migrant children can only occur in a school open to bilingualism.* The reception the deaf children received in a school that respected their language certainly corroborates this stance.

The deaf children learn to use an interpreter and discover new speech situations

Learning to use an interpreter is not necessarily easy, especially for someone who is just barely beginning to speak, as were the children in our class. Only Agnès and Charles, who were the furthest along in their language acquisition, quickly understood that the interpreter was not speaking on her own behalf but merely translating the words exchanged between the teacher and the class.

It took the other children two months to understand this interpretation situation. But they gradually understood, for instance, that it wasn't the interpreter's place to become directly involved in activities with them: she was there only to translate, not to encroach on the teacher's role as instructor and as the person the class should address — deaf children included.

As time went on, the children became accustomed to watching the interpreter and, at the same time, keeping an eye on their teacher's facial expressions so that real communication could develop between them. To make this easier, the interpreter always positioned herself just behind the teacher within the same field of vision. When the teacher explained something using the blackboard, the children had to watch what she was writing or drawing while also following the interpreter's signing, which she always produced as close as possible to the teacher's working space. Understandably, this all required some getting used to on the children's part.

The children also had to learn to use the interpreter when they wanted to say something to the teacher. The following observation shows how comfortable Rémi had become with this arrangement by November 1980. Wanting to tell the teacher about his weekend, he called over the interpreter. She stood behind the teacher who was kneeling in front of him ready for an exchange. Rémi then talked in Sign directly to the teacher, watching her face in order to register her reactions to what he was saying. He also glanced up at the interpreter's lip movements from time to time to make sure that she was interpreting. In other words, Rémi knew exactly how to talk to someone through an interpreter and *maintain perfect eye-contact* in a complex verbal exchange situation.

Besides being vital to the children's ability to participate fully in classroom activities, the interpreter's presence also gave them the chance to experience certain discourse situations they too often missed. When the interpreter translated what was being said between another student and the teacher, they could observe speech spoken around them but not directly to them. As we have seen, this is one of the discourse situations that plays an important role in child language acquisition. The children also experienced, and soon came to understand, being asked questions and given orders as part of the class as a whole.

Besides widening the children's experience of speech, this integration situation (with an interpreter) also allowed them to blossom as individuals. Able to experience what it was like to be part of a fairly large group, the children developed a certain sense of *autonomy* with respect to proposed activities. When a visitor came to observe the interpreting arrangement in the 2nd grade class, it took him over an hour to figure out which four children in the class were deaf! The deaf children were not in any way 'set apart' as a side-group that would parallel what the teacher asked the rest of the class to do. They were among the children addressed by the teacher. It was up to them to follow along or not, to do what she said or not; the teacher was the one to whom they were accountable. Children of their age benefit from pedagogical situations in which they feel treated as *autonomous participants*. This was particularly important for these deaf children who had suffered dearly from an opposite kind of education.

One day when the interpreter was leaving the 2nd grade classroom to join the 1st grade class, Charles called after her and worriedly asked, 'How am I going to understand now?' 'Just watch carefully — you can do it!' she answered. A reassured and attentive expression came back over Charles' face. The interpreter's presence allowed the deaf children to be full participants in their classes, but it was also beneficial for them to gain some autonomy from the interpreter and try to hold their own without her. In these moments without an interpreter they could not catch everything that was said, but they learned to rely on their own mental guesswork. These two situations had to be properly balanced so that the children would feel *very supported* by an environment that adapted to them and their language, and *strongly encouraged* to handle being a deaf person in a hearing environment.

The interpreter noticed a peculiar behavior in the children during recess: not uncommonly, they would interrupt their games to run up and tell her something in Sign and then dash away without waiting for her response. In doing this, they seemed to be reaffirming their own existence as speaking subjects in a situation where some of their verbal communication needs went unsatisfied. Faced with the inevitable verbal frustrations that come with being in a hearing environment — even in play — the children found consolation in the interpreter's mere presence. Their behavior indicated how much they had come to rely on Sign Language as the reference point for their sense of identity.

Because the children's language was acknowledged and they were accepted among the hearing children, they were able to situate themselves and have their place in the hearing school.

A real exchange thus developed between the deaf and hearing children at the crossroads of their mutually respected languages. Every day we observed conversations between deaf and hearing children in which each partner made an effort to speak the other's language.

This was true integration. Through Sign Language, the deaf children were able to take part in everything that was said and experienced at school, and their language was held in high esteem.

We must point out, however, that as the years went by and classroom activities became increasingly focused on academic subjects, having to rely on an interpreter put the deaf children at a disadvantage. No longer could they easily follow what the teacher was showing or writing because they had to watch the interpreter more closely.

What had been possible in the slower-paced early grades, no longer worked in the more advanced grades. Thus, starting with the 1982-83 school year, the deaf children spent their mornings studying academic subjects with a specialized team of teachers while continuing their bilingual class and language activities in the afternoon.

But the children still had their place at school and participated in the extra-curricular activities of the various groups to which they belonged. Most often these integrated activities did not require an interpreter since the deaf and hearing children had learned to meet each other half way, respecting each other's language.

Conclusion: Through Intense Metalingual Activity, the Children Entered into the Two Languages They Were Offered

Embraced as speaking subjects in the bilingual class, the children all developed in a similar way. After rediscovering communication through eye-contact and extra-verbal dialogue, they became interested in speech. They began to acquire speech essentially through extensive play with signifiers in *both* the languages offered them.

At first, speech was for playing, yet in their play the children engaged in very serious identification and 'connecting' activities with their interlocutor. From there, they acquired speech for 'saying', that is, for transmitting a personal content. Through a whole dialectical process involving these two types of speech, the children developed their metalinguistic and referential abilities and gradually entered into each language, respecting its syntactic organization and the modality in which it was spoken.

Such was the path the children followed in acquiring speech. But this is not to say that all six of them progressed 'as one'. Each child came to us with a unique existence linked to a unique set of problems. Although they did seem to go through the same stages in learning to speak, they each went at their own pace and expressed themselves in their own personal way. Incidentally, children never develop in a linear fashion. As Doumic-Girard (1980: 507) writes: 'There are times of progress and there are times of stagnation; and not only are there times of stagnation, there are also times of regression'. We did observe, however, that the children developed similarly as they acquired speech in both of the languages they were offered.

Vocal speech quickly comes to occupy a special place in pedagogy that does not take it as the only goal of deaf education. The primary objective of our educational undertaking was to offer deaf children a *normal communication situation* through Sign Language. Received as complete language-rich beings and acknowledged as different, deaf children become intent on acquiring vocal language, for this is the language through which they identify with their parents and others in their social surroundings. Vocal language even holds a certain fascination for deaf children. They thus give it special attention, provided that proposed activities are offered within *a pedagogy of communication and success based on actively listening to the children themselves.*

The written dimension of vocal language did not escape the children's attention. From the moment they began acquiring speech they also showed keen interest in written language. Our final chapter discusses how these children, recognized as speaking beings, also became literate.

Notes to Chapter 7

1. In the French school system, grades *11ème* and *12ème* respectively.
2. Centre mondial de l'Information sur l'Education bilingue (CMIEB), L'Escalade, 74170 Saint-Gervais, France.

8 Deaf and Literate: The Children's Acquisition of Written Language in the Bilingual Education Program; September 1979–June 1985

Since all classroom interaction revolved around storytelling with illustrated books, the children were exposed to written language right from the moment their speech education began. Chapter 6 described how quickly the children became intrigued with the text they encountered in story books and in the various written-communication situations experienced in class (see page 16).

This chapter will examine how the children acquired written language and began to read and write. First we will briefly analyze the processes involved in acquiring written language as the basis for our approach. Then we will present our work with the children and the results obtained.

How Do Children Acquire Written Language?

In our society, children are exposed to written language well before they enter school. Books and writing usually make up part of their environment from the time they are infants. We often buy storybooks and read them to children even before they can talk. In fact, storytelling is one of the primary settings in which children learn language.

As discussed earlier, language learning varies from one child to the next according to early mother–infant interactions. 'When all goes well' (Winnicott

1960: 591), the good enough mother lavishes language 'lessons' on her child. By creating a space of purposeless play with words not meant to 'say' anything, mothers help their child deal with the awesome realities underlying speech that is meant to say something (see 'A Child's First Words' in Chapter 2, starting on page 65).

Very early, books often become a special part of these fundamental word game activities. Books lend themselves to labeling games and also to storytelling, which satisfies children's need for words spoken simply for their sound, and their equally important need for the contact and aura those sounds create.

Children love to look at storybook images that correspond to words spoken again and again into their ear. Soon they also become interested in what is written next to those images, perhaps realizing that through this graphic representation, they can more fully appropriate those words to which they have become emotionally attached.

Children who are read to acquire quite a collection of words they recognize in books at a very young age. They enjoy 'reading' these words as they reappear page after page in stories they are told. This ability sparks children's interest in writing encountered in their environment — they begin looking for meaning in the written words they see on billboards, in television commercials, on bottle labels, and so on.

In short, reading behaviors are found in young children who are still just acquiring speech.

Learning to write while learning to read

As described above, children become interested in written language even as they are learning to speak. These two modalities of language (written and oral) interrelate in a dialectic favorable to each. Children's ponderings about written language greatly enhance their metalingual activity, which in turn is fundamental to the process of language acquisition. As the language of literature, poetry and pleasing words, written language is the perfect place for playing with language. In our society, learning to speak and read are complementary activities; the process of acquiring language thus encompasses both.

This interrelationship between the acquisition of written and spoken language shows that there is more to learning written language than we generally acknowledge. Just as we never finish learning to speak — never finish emerging as speaking subjects — so we never finish learning to read and write. Even as adults, we are far from able to read everything. There exist books and texts that remain inaccessible to us either because we find their content too foreign, or the language in which they are written too far removed from our own use of language. When both of these factors combine, as they sometimes do, writing can become impenetrable. (This shows that reading involves much more than just deciphering — a point we will discuss later.) Adults' writing activities are often labored, show little variety and are limited to a very restricted number of situations. Yet we could always progress by widening our interaction with written language.

The appropriation of written language, like that of spoken language, is a process that never ends because it is linked to our emerging existence as speaking, reading and writing subjects. But where does this process begin? As in learning to speak (cf. the first three pages of Chapter 6), is there an optimal time when written language learning should begin?

A small number of children learn to read, apparently all on their own, while still acquiring speech — that is, *before* they enter school. It is well known that those children who do not learn to read when they are very young often never fully access written language — even after many years of schooling. The serious problem of scholastic failure now faced in industrialized countries can usually be traced to a poor understanding of written language.

When children are about five years old, they become eager to attend the 'big kids' school. They see this move as a rite of passage to the next generation when they will know how to read and be able to meet the expectations of their parents, for whom attending school primarily means becoming literate.

Yet this is not what happens. At the 'big kids' school, the majority of these children fail in reading even though they looked forward to knowing how. The fact is, their early attraction had more to do with what reading represents — joining the 'grown up' world — than with reading itself. Only those children who already knew how to read — or at least knew a lot about written language — before they entered school succeed scholastically.

Children who become good readers in elementary school are those who talked 'like a book' when they were in kindergarten. They represent one third of all kindergartners. Another third speak much less explicitly and the last third are unable to make themselves understood through speech at all (cf. pp. x and 49–50). These last two thirds are the children who have trouble with reading once they enter elementary school.

As we know, children who have 'trouble learning to read' often continue to think of the world of writing as somewhat foreign for the rest of their lives. 'We are producing a population that gives the appearance of knowing how to read but will never be readers', laments Diatkine (1973: 141).'The phenomenon we are now witnessing will soon require a literacy campaign of a new kind but as urgently needed as in the Third World'. The fact is, reading has very little place in the lives of most schoolchildren. They read neither for pleasure nor to enrich their hearts and minds. In short, they have no access to the culture of the written word.

We have said that the process of learning written language never ends since it is linked to our personal speech history in which we 'become' through language. But for people who don't really have a sense of their own speech, this process remains poorly defined or non-existent. Is it surprising that children who never really had access to speech — speech that would help them find their place in relation to others and the world — are not terribly interested in the world of words and reading?

Something fundamental to the process of learning to read does seem to occur during the period when children acquire speech. The following sections explore what this might be.

The characteristics of written language and the elements of reading

Even though the written word refers to the spoken word, it constitutes a completely different use of language. Written language functions outside of the situation to which it refers. Because of this, words no longer refer to the 'here and now' of an exchange situation. The written word seeks to establish communication outside time and without the presence of an interlocutor. In this modality, words can no longer lean on the context of an utterance   unlike speech, which involves both saying and showing (see the section on 'Speaking is both saying and showing' in Chapter 1). In written language, *everything* must be said and signified through words alone because they are no longer supported by a situation that can be physically seen or experienced by the interlocutor. To function in this way, words must be syntactically organized in a completely different manner from those in oral exchanges, which are linked to a definite situational context. Thus, the belief that written language is a simple transcription of oral language is utterly false, except in very extreme situations such as direct dialogue in novels.

In books, the reader encounters words belonging to his or her language, but finds this language functioning on a particular level, namely that of the narrative. Narrative language is organized according to its own unique syntactic and chronological requirements.

The most commonly used system of graphic transcription is a phonographic one based on a phoneme–grapheme correspondence. We speak of phonographic writing as opposed to ideographic writing ('morphemographic' would actually be the more correct term since these graphic signs denote meaningful linguistic units as opposed to distinctive units such as phonemes). Yet 'no national writing system is the pure incarnation of a single principle or writing procedure' (Ducrot & Todorov, 1979: 197). All of our various written languages have evolved from a combination of these two systems of transcription.

Written European languages are predominantly phonographic, yet also contain important ideographic elements such as orthographic conventions. Spaces between words divide the text into meaningful units of the first articulation, and use-related spellings link these units into lexical series with letters that are unpronounced but which show semantic relationships through visual similarity. Grammatical spellings also employ letters having no phonetic value to indicate gender, number, etc.

This ideographic element in our writing system shows that written language takes both a semantic and a grammatical angle. Together, these perspectives remove the ambiguities of discourse produced without a situational referent and bring out the meaning of the text with the greatest possible clarity. At a psycholinguistic level, the ideographic dimension of written language, as seen in spelling, is 'essentially a matter of reception, that is, reading' (Guion, 1974: 42).

Given these unique characteristics of written language, what does reading actually involve?

Understanding written language, like understanding speech, essentially involves an *act of perception* — in this case visual. The works of Bruner, Bresson and Piaget (1958) on perception show that subjects perceive that which they expect to perceive. Far from remaining passive, subjects actively explore the material at hand by drawing on their knowledge. They thus receive the 'perception of their intellect', in that their intellect determines what will be perceived based on an exploratory strategy of anticipation and verification. Learning to perceive is thus a matter of learning to make a correct hypothesis even if it means going back and collecting more clues when what one chose to perceive proved impertinent.

Speech perception in verbal communication depends on the subject's own intelligent reasoning. This reasoning, in particular, is what makes language intelligible. 'Understanding what another person is saying presupposes productive activity, not passive reception', explains Lentin (1977: 45). Our own verbal process of continual anticipation and verification is what enables us to understand the speech of others.

When we read, our visual perception of a written text involves a similar process: 'The choice to be made — the meaning to attribute to what is perceived

— depends on intelligence ... and on language practice' (Galifret-Granjon, 1966: 470). Practicing language means practicing the narrative and its unique syntactical organization. Only those children who know how to wield language on this level will be capable of anticipating what there is to perceive in text, and thus be able to read. As Eve Malmquist (1973) emphasizes:

> It is, therefore, a complete waste of time to try to teach a child to read until he can articulate clearly and without difficulty. The child must first be able to express his thoughts, to tell stories, or to ask questions in a comprehensible manner. (Malmquist, 1970: 62)

Kindergartners who 'talk like a book' because they have heard their share of stories told over and over again for the pleasure of it, are perfectly ready to perceive this already familiar language in books.

In sum, something fundamental does happen with respect to children's future reading ability when they are just learning to talk. This is the age when, depending on their life experiences, children either do or do not acquire the language of the narrative, that is, the language of writing.

Children who have experienced positive interactions revolving around books are familiar with the use of discourse and language in the world of the written word. They are ready to read what they expect to read. As we have seen, such children already have quite a collection of written words. Through their own metalingual activity, they gradually deduce — *all by themselves* — the phonetic value of various letters as they appear in these familiar written words. Children are able to figure out how to decipher writing because they have already begun to read. In turn, deciphering helps them garner clues to verify their expectations and hypotheses about the meaning of a text. In sum, deciphering isn't an entry into reading but an outcome of it.

Reading is essentially a language activity in which the subject approaches a written text 'expecting meaning' (Hébrard, 1977: 75). The more familiar the subject is with the world of books, and the more easily he or she can manipulate language at that level, the richer this anticipation will be. What then is the key to learning to read?

To read children stories is to teach them to read

Children who truly have access to books and the world of reading 'become good readers and eventually literate persons ... *despite* the experiences to which they have been exposed in school' (Bettelheim, 1982: 9).

Schools completely miss their mark in attempting to teach children to read. This failure can be attributed to an overly utilitarian educational philosophy that primarily emphasized techniques and methods in student reading activities. Such a utilitarian philosophy runs counter to the stated goal, namely, to give all children access to reading.

This propensity to emphasize utilitarian notions is precisely what we have deplored in deaf education. In an overly instrumentalist approach to language, educators present their language to deaf children as though it were merely a code. Consequently, the children produce sentences that would never be heard from the mouth of a hearing child (see pp. 13–16). Deaf children end up 'speaking' while not knowing what speaking is about, which seriously undermines their chances of ever truly gaining access to speech.

To teach reading, schools offer children activities that essentially revolve around deciphering skills. The texts children are given to read are designed primarily to highlight some particular grapheme–morpheme correspondence. For the most part, these 'reader' texts would never be found in any real book because they do not conform, either in form or in content, to the way written language is syntactically organized. In and of themselves, these texts are 'an insult to the child's intelligence' (Bettelheim, 1982: 7).

How can children possibly become aware of the organization of written language and all that writing can convey unless they become familiar with it before they enter school? How can children learn to read, that is, expect meaning from written language, if they have never been exposed to it in the first place? And what good can deciphering skills do for such children? Deciphering is merely a tool for inferring or verifying hypotheses about meaning — hypotheses that only children who have already begun to read are able to make. For children who have not progressed this far, reading is nothing more than a difficult and tedious deciphering exercise. They 'read' *without understanding what reading or writing is about* and without really entering the world of writing and books. They 'read' without becoming readers.

In discussing the shortcomings of schools, Bettelheim (1979: 146) writes: '... it is neither the speed with which knowledge is acquired, nor the propensity for gadgeteering in the laboratories that makes for scientific discoveries. It is curiosity, plus the interest and leisure to follow even idle curiosity, from which flows all deeper understanding'. This holds true for reading as well: children's own curiosity about written language is what enables them to learn to read.

How can this curiosity be fostered in children except by reading and telling them stories? Stories let children experience the endless possibilities that reading can offer by opening the door to literature —'which began as visions of man and was not created to serve utilitarian purposes' (Bettelheim, 1982: 50).

In their desire to share questions that concern adults, children find in literature a world of promise that nourishes their personal lives and imagination. For children, as for adults, literature promises the possibility of better understanding oneself and the world. The imaginary gives implicit meaning to what is real.

What was true in learning to speak, also holds true in learning to read: children need to be told stories (see Chapter 6, pp. 152–166). As seen earlier, children's desire to learn to speak comes from the positive connotations they associate with spoken words through hearing stories that bring meaning to their lives.

A selection of illustrated children's books expose children to the great myths of culture and basic themes of life. The powerful lines and colors in their illustrations also often help exercise children's imagination. When children are read this type of story — 'stories that fascinate them' — they gain an appreciation for written language and want to enter into the 'magic' of reading. They thus try their hardest to succeed. 'In this way the child teaches himself to read' (Bettelheim, 1982: 9).

A case cited by Bettelheim[1] beautifully illustrates the importance of *quality texts* for learning to read. It concerns an American student who attended both a public school and an orthodox Jewish school. At the yeshiva he learned to read the Torah in Hebrew. Although he couldn't speak this language, he was able to translate it perfectly into English. However, when presented with these same passages in English — his mother tongue — he was incapable of reading them: 'he stumbled pathetically over the phonics, and with a grimace exclaimed "I can't"' (Bettelheim, 1982: 55).

'In public school he had been taught to decode laboriously simple English words in meaningless sequences … He knew that no adult could possibly be interested in what he was reading in public school, so he could not work up any interest in it either' (Bettelheim, 1982: 56). By contrast, at the Jewish school, this child was enormously interested in reading the Torah in Hebrew. He had thoroughly applied himself to learning to read and reread bible passages that were meaningful to both himself and adults — who also read them. He realized that, in this context, reading was a productive activity: in an effort to further explore the meaning a passage might hold, something could always be gained from rereading what had already been read.

Reading classic stories to children is the best way to arouse their curiosity about the world of writing. It is also the only way to introduce them to narrative language. Not until children are familiar with this language can they recognize it in books through their own efforts to read.

In conclusion: two examples from literature of very young children who became readers before anyone realized it

In the following passages, Marcel Pagnol (1960) and José Mauro de Vasconcelos (1970) each look back on their childhood and recount how they began to read.

When Pagnol's mother went to market she would leave little three-year-old Marcel in the classroom where his father taught school:

> ... I would sit in the front row, on my best behavior, and admire the paternal omnipotence. In his hand was a bamboo cane: he used it to point out the letters and words he had written on the blackboard and, sometimes, to tap the fingers of a daydreaming dunce.
>
> One morning my mother left me in my usual place and went out without a word, while he wrote on the blackboard in big beautiful letters: 'The mother punished her little boy who had been naughty'.
>
> As he was rounding off an admirable full stop I shouted: 'No! It isn't true!'
>
> My father spun round, stared at me in amazement, and cried: 'What did you say?'
>
> 'Mama didn't punish me! You didn't write down the truth!'
>
> He came up to me.
>
> 'Who said anything about your being punished?'
>
> 'It's written there'.
>
> Surprise left him speechless for a moment.
>
> 'Well, well!' he said at last. 'Can you read?'
>
> 'Yes'.
>
> 'Well, well!' he said again.
>
> He pointed the tip of his bamboo stick at the blackboard. 'All right, read'.
>
> I read the sentence out aloud.
>
> He then picked up a primer and I read out several pages, without any difficulty.
>
> I believe he experienced that day one of the happiest and proudest moments of his life.
>
> When my mother came to fetch me she found me surrounded by four schoolteachers: they had sent their own pupils out into the yard and were

listening to me slowly spelling out the tale of Tom Thumb. But instead of admiring my exploit she grew pale, dropped her parcels, snapped the book shut, and carried me off in her arms, muttering: 'Oh Lord! Oh Lord! ... '

At the door the caretaker, an old Corsican woman, was crossing herself. I learned later that it was she who had gone to fetch my mother, assuring her that 'those gentlemen' were 'bursting' my brain.

At dinner my father affirmed that these were just ridiculous superstitions: I had not exerted myself in any way, I had learned to read as a parrot learns to talk, and he had not even been aware of it.

(Pagnol, 1960: 28–29)

In *My Sweet-Orange Tree*, we meet Vasconcelos at five years old explaining:

I remembered something that had happened the previous week. The family was bewildered. It began when I sat down near Uncle Edmundo at Dindinha's house while he was reading his paper.

'Uncle'.

'What is it, my boy?'

He pulled his glasses to the end of his nose like all grown-up and old people did.

'When did you learn to read?'

'When I was about six or seven years old'.

'Can a person learn to read at five years old?'

'He could. But nobody likes to teach a child who is still so very small',

'How did you learn to read?'

'Like everybody, in the reader. Doing B plus A: BA'.

'Does everybody have to do it that way?'

'All I know of'.

'But really everybody?'

Intrigued, he looked at me.

...

I went around the table and hugged his neck hard. I felt his white hair rub against my forehead very softly.

'That's not for the little horse. I'm going to do something else. I'm going to read'.

'Do you know how to read, Zézé? What story is that? Who taught you?'

'Nobody'.

'That's nonsense'.

I went to the door and said: 'Bring my little horse Friday to see if I can't read ... '

...

'Here's the little horse. Now I want to see'.

He opened the newspaper and showed me a sentence advertising a medicine.

'This product can be found in every pharmacy and specialty shop'.

Uncle Edmundo went to call Dindinha from the yard.

'Mama. He even read *pharmacy* correctly'.

The two of them began to give me things to read and I read them all. My grandmother muttered that the world was lost.

I got the little horse and again hugged Uncle Edmundo. Then he held my chin and told me emotionally, 'You'll go far, you rascal. It wasn't by accident that you were named José. You will be the sun, and the stars will shine around you'.

I kept looking at him without understanding and thinking that he really was nutty.

'You don't understand this. It's the story of Joseph in Egypt. When you get a little bigger I'll tell you the story'.

I loved stories, and the more difficult they were the better I liked them. (Vasconcelos, 1970: 14–19)

When young children are able to read, those around them consider their ability to be extraordinary and even dangerous — allowing little Marcel to read would 'burst his head'. Knowing how to read at a very young age also goes against the established order. ('My grandmother muttered that the world was lost'.) Yet at the same time, this ability to read inspires enormous admiration. Pagnol's father 'experienced that day one of the happiest and proudest moments of his life', and Vasconcelos' uncle declared, 'You will go far, you rascal... You will be the sun, and the stars will shine around you'.

We all know how ecstatic those close to a child are when they hear his or her first words. Discovering that a child knows how to read generates equal excitement — the ability to read is what gives children their full stature as beings of language and communication.

Both Pagnol and Vasconcelos clearly learned to read without anyone — or even themselves — realizing it. Unsettled by the discovery that he could read, José went and questioned his uncle about how, and at what age he had learned to read. But his uncle's response left him perplexed. José knew full well that he himself had not learned to read the alphabet by 'doing B plus A: BA'. When he worriedly asked, 'Does everybody have to do it that way?' his uncle didn't know quite how to respond. As we know, deciphering is *not* the key to reading. These two children learned to read at such a young age because they were immersed in the oral language of stories and fairy tales: little Marcel had a school teacher for a father, and José had an uncle who quenched his thirst for tales. ('I loved stories, and the more difficult they were the better I liked them'.)

Under such conditions children learn to read all by themselves. Their love for stories draws them into the world of writing and leads them to discover, from their still limited ability to read, that deciphering is a useful tool that can shift their reading ability into high gear ('The two of them gave me things to read and I read them all'.) Such deciphering is possible only when children have already begun to read.

Because reading is essentially a language activity, it falls well within the processes of language acquisition and can be acquired almost naturally. Yet 'acquired naturally' does not mean 'taken for granted'. Quite to the contrary, these naturally acquired abilities can develop only through a privileged relationship with an adult whose responses are on a level with the child's questions and interests. This requires certain 'luxury conditions' similar to those required for speech acquisition (cf. page 144).

In light of the principles presented above, we will now show how our storytelling-based bilingual class offered the children every opportunity to interact with and acquire written language as they were learning to speak.

How We Worked with the Children in the Bilingual Education Program to Enable Them to Acquire Written Language

When the children were just barely beginning to speak and their linguistic activity still revolved primarily around playing with signifiers, the written texts they encountered during storytelling gave them added opportunity to play with language. The children derived great satisfaction from knowing the written representation of whatever words they were learning. During storytelling, they would point to these words as they appeared on the pages of the story being told, and take advantage of these written representations as a pretext for repeating the words in Sign Language or in vocal language.

Written language thus served as a catalyst for the children's metalinguistic activity. This visual and permanent representation of language was also a mirror in which they could contemplate their ability to perceive language as an object to be studied — a realization that brought them great satisfaction.

To respond to this interest in written language, we would select two or three sentences from passages that had particularly touched the children during the story, and print them largely and clearly on the blackboard (matching the print the children saw in books). We offered this writing to the children as a gift, and each read the sentences in our own language — the deaf teacher in Sign Language and the hearing teacher in vocal language. The children then used the written text for various recognition and evocation activities that further encouraged their manipulation and acquisition of each language (cf. Chapter 6, pp. 161–166).

The children were delighted when they realized that writing could recreate a particular utterance that had been spoken during storytelling.

It wasn't long before their curiosity about writing evolved further. Parallel to their intense play with signifiers, the children also began to acquire speech for the purpose of telling about themselves and transmitting content of their own. At this point, they began searching written texts not just for known content but also for unknown content. The children became interested in all the different kinds of written text they found around them, and would try to figure out what these writings meant.

Starting in January and February 1981, the children became keenly interested in all written communication situations experienced in class. For instance, when Linda received an invitation from one of her hearing classmates, she eagerly opened it and tried to figure out by herself the message contained on the card. She recognized the name of her friend, *Marie*, and the words *petits* (little), *amis* (friends) and *mercredi* (Wednesday) in the note that read: *Marie recevra ses petits amis mercredi prochain à partir de 15h30* (Marie will receive her little friends next Wednesday at 3:30 p.m.). All on her own Linda had grasped the essence of the message, yet was happy to have an adult read it to her to confirm what she herself had read. In this way she obtained the remaining information that had escaped her.

Another child, Sabine, was curious about what was written in books that had not been told in class. She would go to the library and pick out a simple book with clear illustrations and amply spaced, repetitive text. Then she would begin 'reading' it by translating all the written words she knew into signs. For every word she did not know, she would sign IMPOSSIBLE. Sabine knew exactly what she could and could not read. Then she would ask whichever adult was present to tell her in Sign the meaning of each word she did not know. Having obtained these explanations she would resume her reading with great interest, exuding both contentment and pride. It made Sabine happy that she could identify with her teachers who knew how to read stories to children. She seemed to be motivated by the same sense of fascination that Jean Paul Sartre (1964: 46–48) speaks of in recounting childhood memories about his mother reading him a story: '... I realized: it was the book that was speaking ... I then became jealous of my mother and resolved to take her role away'.

To respond to the interest and curiosity the children demonstrated toward written language while still just acquiring speech, we began proposing various receptive and expressive writing activities, namely reading texts, dictating to adults, and making written utterances.

Reading texts

Once a story had been told by each teacher in her own language, the hearing teacher would write, on a large piece of paper, a text that closely followed and summarized the storyline. At first we wrote these texts in the present tense. For example, to open Anderson's tale, 'The Nightingale', we wrote: 'In the forest next to the emperor's castle lives a very beautiful bird'.

After a few months of having the children read such texts, we began to introduce stories in the traditional manner with 'Once upon a time ...' For instance, for the story of Goldilocks we wrote:

> *Il était une fois une petite fille qui s'appelait Boucle d'Or et qui habitait avec sa maman une maisonnette près du bois.*

(Once upon a time there was a little girl named Goldilocks who lived in a little house near the woods with her mother.)

We then let the story unfold in a sophisticated interweaving of the imperfect and simple past tenses. For example, when Goldilocks is lost in the woods:

> *... elle marchait, elle marchait quand elle aperçut à travers les arbres une très jolie maison.*

(... she had been walking and walking when she noticed a very pretty house through the trees.)

Over time we also lengthened the texts considerably. Rather than summarizing the story we transcribed it nearly in full. Each day we added a bit more text and noted, 'to be continued'. By the end of the week we would complete the story and close it with 'The End'. These texts were the basis for the following three activities:

(1) Discovering the text with the hearing teacher

Given a text, the children tried to understand it on their own by helping each other. The teacher did not intervene except to help with problems or to point out a particular ideographic marker that was fundamental to understanding the text. In this way we helped the children develop an implicit knowledge of grammar, without which reading would be impossible. For instance, we would explain the ideographic value of letters that marked notions of gender and number and that established grammatical relationships between words.

During such group readings the children exercised their metalinguistic abilities at a lexical or morphological level as well as at a grammatical level. When they came across a word they had never seen, they hypothesized about its meaning in light of the story they already knew. For example, when they first encountered the word *propriétaire* (proprietor, owner), one child guessed its meaning based on the context and jumped up to get a text that had been studied several months earlier. He then flipped through it to find the word *propriété* (property). All on his own, he had realized that words can be grouped into families. When faced with the expression *s'écrier* (to cry out, exclaim), the children noticed that it contained the verb *crier* (to cry, call out, shout) along with a pronominal construction, and realized that this was like a pair of verbs they knew well: *s'appeler* (to be called) and *appeler* (to call). And when the children came across the sentence, *Ils sortirent de la maison* (they left the house), they noticed the plural markers and deduced that the *ils* must refer to the three bears in the story. In sum, the children enjoyed finding grammatical markers themselves and explaining them the way the teacher did. Through this regular behavior, they fully internalized orthographical rules and written structures. For instance, when they came to the expression, *Je peux vous aider* (I can help you), one child noted the *er* ending, which is required on any verb that directly follows another verb. This observation led the children to realize that the pronoun *vous* did not refer to several people but to the old woman to whom the heroine was speaking. This is how they discovered the polite *vous* form for 'you'.

The children sometimes confused words that were very similar such as *nuage* and *neige* (cloud, snow), and *dessert* and *désert* (dessert, desert). But they quickly learned to reject their mistaken reading hypotheses when they did not fit the general meaning of the text. Such confusion between words showed that the children had acquired considerable knowledge about writing but still needed to refine what they knew by more closely analyzing the material to be perceived. Having started with a fairly global approach to reading, the children gradually adopted a more analytical approach.

As developed by the children, this was a true reading activity. They 'expected to find meaning' in a written text. Because the children were told the story first, they were able to anticipate what they would be reading, and this ability encouraged them in their investigative strategy of anticipating and verifying what they perceived. In short, they proceeded like scientists, building on their own ability to read by pursuing their *quest for meaning*. As the children confirmed what they knew and acquired new knowledge, they internalized written language in ever deeper ways.

During this time devoted to uncovering the text's meaning, child-child and child-teacher interactions happened in all forms — vocal French, signed French, mime, Sign Language. But the second reading was done exclusively in Sign Language.

(2) Reading the text with the deaf teacher

The deaf teacher would go through the entire text again sentence by sentence, translating it into Sign Language. First she signed at a normal pace, then went back and signed in slow motion. Next, the children were each invited to point out, directly on the written sentence, those written words that corresponded to the Sign Language sentence as it was being produced. Thus, for the written sentence, *ils sortent de la maison* (they leave the house), the children pointed to the words in the following order: *la maison, ils, de, sortent*. This was the order that corresponded to the Sign Language sentence in which MAISON appeared first. Then came the classifier for three people (representing the three bears), signed where the non-dominant hand still remained in place from signing MAISON. The sign SORTIR then began from that same point (a marker having the same grammatical value as the preposition 'from') and was carried through to complete the sentence. Again, this was all done in slow motion in order to highlight elements of placement and directionality that simultaneously affected the execution of a sign. This enabled the children to match the various gestural parameters with the corresponding words in the written French sentence.

Such matching exercises required a very refined and sophisticated analysis of the grammatical structure of each language being compared. In fact, the children were not the only ones who proceeded like linguists; the teachers delved into serious linguistic analyses as well.

In order to translate a text into Sign Language and divide signed sentences into meaningful units, the deaf teacher had to reflect intently on her own language. She also took advantage of what came to light during the children's first approach to the text with the hearing teacher. The deaf teacher wielded Sign Language beautifully but did not have full command of written French. (Until our class, no deaf person in France had enjoyed this kind of bilingual pedagogy in learning to read.) Similarly, the hearing teacher's French was very strong (she composed the texts) but she did not know Sign Language well enough to ensure a good translation of the texts into that language.

To accomplish these *translation* and *matching* exercises between the two languages, the teachers had to collaborate closely. Incidentally, the children were very attentive to discussions between the teachers in this area.

Let us take another example:

Dans la forêt, le petit chaperon rouge rencontre le loup qui lui dit *«Je sais où est la maison de ta grand-mère».*

(In the forest, Little Red Ridinghood encountered the wolf, *who said to her*, 'I know where your grandmother's house is',)

In this sentence, the sign DIT (said) was varied in two of its parameters. First, the position of the signer shifted to where the sign LOUP was just made. This shift served to indicate who would be speaking, just as *qui* did in French. Second, the movement of the sign was directed downward to show that the wolf was addressing Little Red Ridinghood, who was smaller than himself. In French, this same indication was given by the pronoun *lui*. Again, the deaf teacher signed slowly, highlighting all these parameters so that the children could match them to elements in the French sentence. In this way, it became clear to the children that *qui* referred to the wolf, and *lui* to Little Red Ridinghood.

In a sentence such as,

Elle marchait, elle marchait, quand tout à coup elle aperçut une très jolie maison.

(She had been walking and walking when suddenly she noticed a very pretty house.)

the gestural variations on the signs MARCHER (to walk) and APERCEVOIR (to notice) helped the children firmly grasp the imperfect and simple past verbal tenses. For instance, when MARCHER was signed in a repeated movement with the cheeks puffed out, the children pointed to the imperfect *ait* ending on the French verb.

Only through this detailed comparison with Sign Language could we be sure that the children understood the written text perfectly in all its nuance and without any remaining uncertainties.

Reading the text in signed French would have inevitably led to contradictions and confusion. Signs produced in French word order lose their inflectional variations and no longer follow the *logical syntax* of a gestural language that is organized in terms of *space*.

On a par with Sign Language, deaf children are able to grasp its syntactical organization — and thus the grammatical categories of language — without limitation. Once they easily manipulate these notions in a visual language, deaf children are then able to transpose them into French syntax.

In matching Sign Language with written French, the children closely analyzed each language. A person cannot become a reader without approaching language grammatically. For deaf children, such an approach is not fully possible without passing by way of Sign Language — this is a *necessary* step.

Once the children had perfectly understood the text, it then became the basis for a variety of vocal speech activities.

(3) Using reading as a support for vocal speech

This activity took place with the hearing teacher. She would read the text out loud, dividing it into small word groups for the children to read on her lips and then repeat aloud. The children looked at the text only when preparing to speak, not when actually vocalizing.

The support of written text seemed to free the children from the work of constructing their utterance and allow them to give their undivided attention to controlling their articulatory movements. Their familiarity with the phonetic and ideographic value of letters and groups of letters in particular contexts also helped them control their articulation. The children were able to benefit from deciphering the text because they already knew how to read. In fact, knowing how to read is what enabled them to decipher text. The permanence of writing also aided the children in vocalizing by allowing them to go back over words and sentences as many times as they wished.

Since the children were already completely comfortable with the content of the text, having read it several times in each language, they were delighted to then read it several times out loud. They were able to do so with proper intonation, which showed that they had fully integrated the meaning of the text and its syntactic structures.

All of these reading activities made the children want to learn to write. We thus gave them the opportunity to experience various writing situations.

Dictating to an adult

As a gift to the children, we would write down whatever each child wanted us to. In addition to placing great value on their budding attempts at personal expression, this also gave them the satisfaction of having some writing that was completely personal and all their own. Taking dictation for the children eventually became a regular activity which, borrowing from Clesse (1977), we called *la dictée à l'adulte*. Everything the children dictated to an adult was kept in their own special notebook, which they called their 'notebook of private stories'.

The children cherished their notebooks. Often it was the first thing they showed their parents when they arrived home, and the first thing they presented to us in the morning if their parents had added something new. One morning, even before saying hello, Linda showed us her notebook. She pointed out that her mother had added the word 'Sonia' to the sentence we had written the day before: *Mon amie ... habite au cinquième étage* (my friend .... lives on the fifth floor). At the time, Linda had been unable to make us understand the name of her friend.

This dictation activity began at a time when the children were still just beginning to speak and their verbal abilities remained limited. They tended to address the deaf teacher since she was the one best able to understand what they were trying to say. She would reformulate each child's statement into correct Sign Language. Then the hearing teacher would translate it into French and write it down in the child's notebook.

Once the children's speaking abilities had improved, they started addressing the hearing teacher directly when they wanted to say something fairly simple. We observed that these were the instances when children's 'simultaneously signed and vocalized' utterances most closely followed vocal language syntax. For example, when Agnès dictated a story to the hearing teacher, she would use a vocally articulated *je* (I) while pointing to herself. In Sign Language this pronominal marker would not have appeared except as an inflectional variation on the direction of the verb. Agnès was clearly resorting to a French grammatical construction.

Over time the children's stories became longer and more complicated: One child told us about a broken car windshield and how the insurance would pay for it! (Sign Language allowed the children to talk about all sorts of things.) Dictation thus offered the children rich experiences with written language; and because these writings referred to their own lives, they were all the easier to memorize.

Yet giving dictation to an adult did not satiate the children's desire to produce writing themselves. Thus, it wasn't long before we proposed a third activity in which they wrote their own utterances.

The written utterance

In January 1982, after the children had been reading texts and giving dictation to adults for one year, we started the new activity of making written utterances. The children were not left on their own in this personal writing exercise, but guided and supported pedagogically so they could truly learn to write.

The activity unfolded in the following manner. Once a story was fully appreciated and savored, having been told and read several times in each language, we invited each child to tell us which passage had touched him or her the most. Delighted to be asked about the story and invited to express their feelings, the children would leaf through the book, reflect, and finally decide upon their choice. We then asked them to share their choice with the deaf teacher, who would correctly reformulate their utterance for them. The hearing teacher would then translate it into vocal language, having each child recognize on her lips the utterance he or she had chosen to produce. Only then were the children invited to write down their special utterance by themselves.

For this independent writing exercise, we explained to the children that if they did not know how to write a word, they were free to look it up in familiar books or in the often read texts available to them.

A very special atmosphere of serious and absorbing occupation would fall over the classroom as the children happily began looking among texts and books for the words they needed. Astoundingly, the children knew exactly which book or text contained the word they needed. In one instance, a child chose to write *le cheval rencontre le vieux chameau* (the horse meets the old camel). He was unsure how to write the word *rencontre*, and it did not appear in the text of the story about the old camel and the horse. So he went to the corner where we kept stories that had already been told and without a moment's hesitation picked out a story told over a year earlier about some animals that went looking for summer. He opened right to the page that began with: *De l'autre côté de la rivière, il rencontra un beau bélier aux cornes recourbées* (From the other side of the river he met a beautiful ram with curled horns). He then wrote from memory the word he had found. For this child, there was a strong connection between the word *rencontre* and this tale about a string of encounters.

This was perfectly regular behavior for the children. They were very confident in their ability to find the words they needed to construct their writing. This shows that storytelling provided the children with a highly structured and ritualized framework that helped them memorize language in both its oral and written forms.

It was not unusual for the children to help each other during this activity. For example, one child wanted to write the word *voyage* but didn't know where to find it. The child to whom he turned immediately retrieved the book *Helen, la petite fille du silence et de la nuit* (Helen, The Little Girl of Silence and Darkness) and opened to this page:

Helen voyagea beaucoup, elle alla dans tous les pays pour expliquer qu'il fallait s'occuper des enfants sourds et aveugles.

(Helen traveled a lot; she went to every country to explain that people should attend to deaf and blind children.)

Another child, observing this exchange, went and found the book *Histoire d'un arbre* (Story of a Tree), which begins:

Durant toute la nuit, l'arbre rêva qu'il partait pour un long voyage.

(All night long, the tree dreamt that he was leaving for a long trip.)

The children were keenly aware of what they did and did not know how to write. They did not bother to check words they were sure of, but looked up the rest in books and texts. These were words they were able recognize but had not yet memorized or expressed in writing themselves.

The children thus experienced the fact that a person cannot invent, but rather has to learn how words are written. And learn they did. Through their own observations and research using a corpus of written language with which they were familiar, the children acquired the syntax and orthographical elements of written French. Here again, the children were the primary builders and organizers of their own knowledge; our pedagogical objective was essentially to encourage their manipulation of written language as much as possible.

As we have seen, a reader cannot effectively read without fully taking into account the information provided by grammatical and usage-related spellings. Both are essential to decoding meaning and thus to reading itself. The fact that we can only read what we expect to perceive means, in effect, that we can read only what we would be capable of writing ourselves. For this reason, the results of the children's written language appropriation will be presented through an analysis of texts that they themselves produced.

In our view, the only true way to test a subject's reading level is to analyze his or her ability to write, both in terms of *organizing* the narrative and *respecting orthographical rules*. Our analysis of the children's writings will thus focus on these two areas.

Results: The Children's Writings from January 1982 to June 1985

Over time, all the children showed a similar development in their writings. Here we will track this development through examples taken almost exclusively from our youngest student, Agnès, who benefited the earliest from bilingual education.

When the children first began producing written utterances in the manner just described, their writings closely followed the original text, faithfully rendering some element of the story. In connection with *Little Red Ridinghood*, for instance, Agnès (who was 7;1 years old at the time) wrote:

Le petit chaperon s'en va dans la forêt elle arrive chez sa mère grand: «moi le petit chaperon j'apporte galette dorée.»

(Little ridinghood sets off into the forest she arrives at her grandmother's: 'me little ridinghood I bring golden cake'.)
(April 1982)

It was not long, however, before the children began to take liberties with the story as told. They invented details, often drawn from illustrations in the storybook. Sometimes they even reversed the roles of various characters. In connection with the tale *La plus mignonne des petites souris* (The cutest little mouse), Agnès wrote:

mignonne souris cueille des fleurs dans jardin.

(cute mouse picks flowers in garden.)
(June 1982)

No such detail exists in this story about a papa mouse's extraordinary search to find a very powerful husband for his cute daughter. He even takes off in a helicopter to ask the sun if he will marry her. Agnès, touched by how cute this mouse is, portrays her picking flowers just like two other very familiar characters — Goldilocks and Little Red Ridinghood. For this same tale, Patrick, who was fascinated by the helicopter trip, wrote a sentence based on one of the illustrations in the story book:

la vache voit un hélicoptère.

(the cow sees a helicopter.)

The children's tendency to stray from the original story led them to write their own original stories based on the one they were told. Here is one such text written by Agnès:

Piro joue avec le vrai chien dans le jardin. Piro prend le chien et il l'assit sur la balançoire.

(Piro plays with the real dog in the garden. Piro takes the dog and sits him on the swing.)
(March 1983)

In the original story, Piro is very sad because all he has is stuffed dogs. Agnès invented the part about putting the dog on the swing, apparently inspired by the poetic tale, *Une petite fille sur une balançoire* (A little girl on a swing), told in June 1981. The next day, in connection with the same story, Agnès wrote:

> *Piro entre chez le chef des pompiers pour lui demander: «je veux deux oeufs au chocolat.»*

(Piro goes into the chief fireman's office to ask him: 'I want two chocolate eggs'.)

On her paper next to the date, Agnès noted, *bientôt paque* (Easter soon). In the actual story, Piro does in fact call upon firemen, with their aura of power, to satisfy his desire to have a real dog. In her own story, Agnès picks up, but transposes, the theme of turning to firemen to satisfy a deep desire. Agnès was just turning eight years old and was enraptured with the idea of Easter and chocolate eggs. In fact at Easter time a year later, she wrote a long, original story in which a helicopter drops chocolates on Easter day.

The children's stories tended to be longer whenever they involved this type of self-expression. Here are two examples from Agnès' writings in 1984:

> *Célestine mit sa belle robe blanche et elle se coiffa avec deux noeuds assortis à son parapluie rose.*
> *Mais, Ernest ne voulut pas d'aller chez le photographe. Célestine lui dit: «c'est dommage !»*

> (Célestine put on her beautiful white dress and fixed her hair with two bows that matched her pink umbrella.
> But, Ernest did not want to go to the photographer's. Célestine said to him: 'that's a pity!')
> (January 1984)

In this first example, Agnès reproduces a very satisfying, narcissistic scene (putting on a beautiful dress) presented in the story, but follows it with a frustrating scene that departs from the original storyline (in which Ernest responds positively to Célestine's request that he have his picture taken). Born deaf, Agnès had experienced enormous frustration in her attempts to communicate until a relatively advanced age. Moreover, as the oldest of three children, she often experienced situations in which her desires went unsatisfied for lack of time or money. In fact, in later texts, she often alluded to money.

The second example comes from Agnès' writings in connection with *Le petit loir est très content* — a story based on 'The Grasshopper and the Ant' but organized in a repetitive format in which four animals (a mouse, a bird, a dragonfly and a cricket) come knocking at the dormouse's door:

> *Un petit loir, une souris, un oiseau et une libellule font le ménage dans*

la maison du petit loir.

   Ils rient et danser.

   Un soir, le petit loir entend frapper à sa porte et une petite voix lui cria: «C'est moi, le chat, il fait froid dehors, laisse-moi entrer dans ta maison si chaud et si proprette.»

   Le petit loir lui répond: «Mais toi, n'as fait que boire le lait dans son bol.»

   Mais, le petit loir est bon coeur.

   Il lui répond: «bon, tu peux venir chez moi, mais tu nettoieras le plancher.»

   Le chat lui répond: «Oui, d'accord.»

(A little dormouse, a mouse, a bird and a dragonfly are cleaning up in the house of the little dormouse.

They laugh and to dance.

One evening, the little dormouse hears knocking at his door and a little voice cries out to him: 'It's me, the cat, it's cold outside, let me come into your house that is so warm and so tidy'.

The little dormouse answers him: 'But you, only drank the milk in its bowl'.

But the little dormouse is good heart.

He answers him: 'fine, you can come into my house, but you will clean the floor'.

The cat answers him: 'Yes, OK'.)

(May 1984)

Agnès opens her story with the first three animals of the story already safe in the dormouse's house. The fourth animal she introduces, however, is not a cricket, but a cat — an animal she wanted very much to have.

The more the children expressed themselves in their texts, the more they began writing original pieces that no longer showed any connection to the story upon which they were based. For instance, given the story *Ernest et Célestine vont pique-niquer* (Ernest and Célestine go for a picnic), Agnès, now 9;9 years old, wrote the following:

   Il était une fois, un gros ours qui s'appelait Ernest, il y avait un grand jardin d'Ernest qui vivait très heureux.

   Il voyait toujours des petites souris qui venaient dans sa jardin et tous les petites souris se adoraient jouer dans la jardin d'Ernest.

   Quand, tous les enfants allaient dans leur maison et Ernest leur donnait à chacun des bonbons.

   Un jour, une petite fille demanda à Ernest: «Je perdue mes parents !»

   Ernest eut une bonne idée et il lui réponda: «tu reste avec moi pour

toujours, tu auras une vivre très heureux avec moi!» la fille lui dit: «Merci
beaucoup, tu es gentil.»

Un jour la petite fille dit à Ernest: «Je n'ai pas de nom, est ce que tu
peux me donner le nom pour moi ?» Ernest lui réponda: «Je donne le nom
pour toi: Célestine» et elle lui dit: «Je te remercie.» Puis, ils vivaient très
heureux !!!

(Once upon a time, a big bear who was named Ernest, there was a big
garden of Ernest who lived very happily.

He always saw little mice who came in his garden and all the little
mice adored themselves playing in Ernest's garden.

When, all the children went into their house and Ernest gave each one
of them candy.

One day, a little girl asked Ernest: 'I lost my parents!'

Ernest had a good idea and he answered: 'you stay with me forever,
you will have a very happy life with me!' the girl said: 'Thank you very
much, you are nice'.

One day the little girl said to Ernest: 'I don't have a name. can you
give me the name for me?' Ernest answered: 'I give you the name for
you: Célestine' and she said: 'Thank you'. Then, they were living very
happily!!!)
(January 1985)

In this story, nothing remains of the original tale except the names of the
characters — Ernest and Célestine — and Ernest's identity as a nice big, protective bear with whom life is pleasant. Célestine, a very humanized mouse in the
original story, becomes a little girl in Agnès'. This clearly shows the projection
mechanisms at work in Agnès' reading of the stories.

In this text, Agnès alludes to her own life experiences. But significantly, she
does so by drawing on situations presented in stories she particularly enjoyed.
The theme of Ernest's garden being a place where mice can play, for instance,
comes from the tale of 'The Selfish Giant', by Oscar Wilde. This story — told
four months earlier — is about a giant who forbids children from entering his
very lovely garden. The giant then has a change of heart, becomes the children's
friend and welcomes them into his garden. Similarly, the theme of a little girl
without a name comes directly from a story we told a year and a half earlier.

Such references show how much storytelling nourished the children's
imaginations and personal lives, and thus developed their capacity for true self-
expression.

The little girl whom Agnès introduces in this story has lost her parents. The
children often encountered this theme in the stories they were told. But when we

told the story of Hansel and Gretel in December 1983, Agnès expressed how upset she was that parents could want to lose their child in the forest and show such utter rejection of their children. This was not how Agnès reacted when a child got lost in the forest by him or herself, such as in Goldilocks. In Agnès' text the little girl is rejected to the extent that she does not have a name, an existence, or recognition from anyone. As a composite of two good characters (the protective bear and the giant who becomes a friend to children), the bear who gives the girl a name is doubly invested with positive connotations. Finally, in giving this story a happy ending, Agnès demonstrates her ability to create healing situations.

As the children began expressing themselves in very deep ways in their stories, we noticed a particular recurring theme in the writings of each child.

Agnès' writings often brought up the theme of *names* and linked it to the issue of children being accepted or rejected by their parents. In February 1985, we told a basically humorous story about a tortoise who decided to get out and see the world but never managed to get started. Drawing from that story, Agnès wrote quite a tragic text about some parents who

> *...ne peuvent pas faire d'enfant; mais un beau jour, (de) la maman est née une petite tortue toute verte, on l'appelait la «tortue verte», mais le papa n'est pas d'accord, il voulait donner un nom «tortue léon». Mais la maman ne voulait pas de ce prénom, elle préfère: «Tortuléon».*

(...couldn't have any children; but one fine day, (of) the mother was born a little, completely green tortoise, it was called the 'green tortoise', but the daddy didn't agree, he wanted to give a name 'tortoise leon'. But the mommy did not want this first name, she preferred: 'Tortoiseleon'.)

Agnès goes on to describe the tortoise's transformation into a chameleon and how his parents reacted to this change:

> *...ils se disaient: c'est bête que on fait l'enfants.*

(...they would say to each other: it's stupid that we make the childs.)

The mother does not give her baby tortoise a name. When the father suggests they give him the name 'Leon', the mother transforms the name into a combination of two animal names: tortoise and chameleon. This new combined name clearly disturbs the baby's very existence — he changes into a chameleon. In this way, Agnès forcefully expresses all the ambivalence that can surround the desire to have a child. She also describes the child's feelings of rejection resulting from the parent's battle over what to name him and from their final conclusion (i.e. 'it's stupid that we make the childs'). In her story, the child does not survive this situation very well.

One week later, in connection with a story about some parents who wanted boys but always had girls, Agnès wrote a story along the same lines about some parents who wanted a girl but had a boy:

> *Les parents sont mécontents... La maman eut une bonne idée et elle dit à papa: «il ne faut pas donner de prénom au garçon parce qu'ils n'aimaient pas ce garçon.»*

(The parents were unhappy... The mama had a good idea and she said to papa: 'the boy must not be given a name because they didn't like this boy'.)

Here, Agnès clearly expresses the decision not to name a child as a clear sign of rejection. But the story continues — a second baby is born (Agnès' texts were getting longer and longer):

> *c'est une fille mais la maman ne veut pas la garder.*

(it's a girl but the mama doesn't want to keep her.)

This girl does not receive a name either. Then:

> *Un jour, les parents leur donnèrent les prénoms d'animal... pour l'aîné: l'éléphant, pour le deuxième: la chatte. mais les deux enfants l'ont su et les parents ont changé d'avis, alors ils donnèrent pour l'aîné: Thomas, pour la deuxième Virginie. La famille fut très heureuse et vécurent pour toujours.*

(One day, the parents gave them animal names... for the eldest: the elephant, for the second: the cat. but the two children found out and the parents changed their minds, so they gave for the eldest: Thomas, for the second Virginia. The family was very happy and lived forever.)

Agnès gives her story a happy ending: The children feel intolerably rejected when they find out they have been given animal names; but their reaction makes the parents change their mind. By naming their children, the parents finally acknowledge and accept them.

Agnès' texts reflect the thought she gave to the importance of naming. Naming grants children their status as subjects and as acknowledged speaking beings having a rightful place in the world. Agnès' approach is even more moving when we consider that she did not know she had a name until she was four and a half years old and learned of it through Sign Language. Her parents had indeed given her a name, but it never reached her through oral language. This is the case for many deaf children.

The *content* of the children's texts showed that they had been produced in a true act of writing. In and through these writings the children developed themes of thought to better understand themselves and the world, thus approaching writing in the same way they approached reading.

But what *form* did these stories take? Agnès' January 1985 text about Ernest and Célestine (transcribed above in full), demonstrates that Agnès knew how to *organize* a story: First she presents the characters, next recounts a progression of events, and finally concludes with a denouement in perfect fairy tale style. The verb tenses she uses are those of a narrative and show a perfect command of when to use the imperfect versus the simple past. Only in her last sentence does she misuse the imperfect. The sentence should read *Puis ils vécurent très heureux* (Then, they lived very happily). By 9th March Agnès was able to correctly use this irregular simple past form of the verb *vivre* (see text cited above).

Agnès' January 1985 text does not contain a single *spelling or grammar* error even though she took only about ten minutes to write it and did not bother to check the spelling of any word in available books. Her only errors are ones of misuse. For example, she mistakenly treats *souris* as a masculine noun in *tous les petits souris*, after properly handling it as a feminine noun in the previous line (*des petites souris*). Her error was one of performance, not competence.

When the children wrote about things that truly preoccupied them, they became entirely absorbed in expressing content and sometimes let a few superficial errors slip through. This can happen to anyone in writing a text that requires a lot of attention to content. We have to reread what we've written in order to catch our mistakes. In the children's case, all we had to do was underline their errors — the children almost always knew how to make the corrections themselves. In the above text, for instance, Agnès wrote *réponda* instead of *répondit*. This was a performance error, probably brought on by the verb form *demanda* just before it. Agnès had correctly used *répondit* in much earlier texts that didn't involve her nearly as personally.

We observed that the children's texts contained fewer errors the more closely they followed the original story, and the easier they were to construct. As the above examples show, these texts were often written without a single mistake. The mistakes we did find attested to the children's strong command of orthographical rules. The children's occasional errors revealed what they were thinking at the time. For instance, in mistakenly adding the feminine *e* to the end of *perdu* in *Je perdue mes parents!* (I lost my parents!), Agnès highlights the fact that it was a little girl who had suffered this fate.

We might point out that the children's spelling was always impeccable, even when it came to words that might appear difficult, such as *cueille* and *balançoire* in the above-quoted texts.

Taught according to the pedagogy we offered, the children showed no trouble spelling, either in terms of grammar rules or accepted spellings. We did not encounter any of the spelling disorders frequently found in hearing children. The cause of massive failures in spelling and grammar lies not with children but with those who teach them.

The *content*, *organization*, and *orthographical form* of the children's writings showed that the children were indeed becoming literate. The children saw written language as a place where, through reading and writing, they could delve deeper into answering their questions about themselves and the world.

Conclusion: Offered a Bilingual Education in Which They Were Recognized as Speaking Beings, the Children Also Became Literate Beings

Through truly experiencing literature, the children appropriated written language. In the bilingual setting we offered the children, they gained access to the world of books as soon as they began to speak. They did so through Sign Language — a language in which they knew no handicap either in accessing language or in entering the world of fairy tales and stories.

The children in our class experienced the natural language-acquisition situation created by storytelling. Their curiosity about the writing they encountered in books greatly contributed to their metalinguistic development: learning to read meant learning to speak with ever greater precision in the two languages offered them.

The children concomitantly entered into three different worlds of language: *Sign Language*, *vocal language in its oral form*, and *vocal language in its written form*. Deaf children's access to oral vocal communication remains limited because of the sensorial barrier of deafness — for instance, they cannot speechread vocal speech unless it is addressed to them directly. Yet allowed the opportunity to appropriate written language through Sign Language, these same children need not experience any limitation in written communication. However, any real and in-depth appropriation of written language requires meticulous, well-thought-out translation work between the two languages in both reading and writing activities. Figure 8.1 illustrates the resulting bilingual situation experienced by the children.

Accessing written language not only helped the children understand themselves better and situate themselves in relation to others and the world (just as accessing speech does), it also helped them to situate themselves in relation to the two languages encountered. As the children acquired written language, they quickly began to translate what they read into Sign Language. In their eyes, it was inappropriate and even comical to do a word-for-word translation into signed French. (Signed French simply does not conform to the syntactical organization of a visual-gestural language.) This attitude was an indication of the

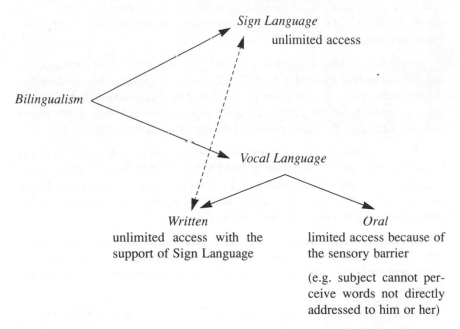

Sign Language
unlimited access

Bilingualism

Vocal Language

Written
unlimited access with the support of Sign Language

Oral
limited access because of the sensory barrier

(e.g. subject cannot perceive words not directly addressed to him or her)

FIGURE 8.1

children's ability to move between two languages. As they acquired written language, their bilingualism became increasingly intentional and well-defined.

The results obtained show that the children were able to become readers and writers through a very unique pedagogy that relied solely on Sign Language. No deciphering techniques were used. In the other direction, however, familiarity with writing helped the children enormously in their acquiring vocal speech. The permanence of writing allowed them to return as many times as they wished to sentence structures or words they wanted to practice vocally.

By confirming that deciphering is not a preliminary step to reading, our research on written language acquisition in deaf children has very specific implications for the teaching of reading in regular schools.

In previous chapters we showed that in order to appropriate vocal language, deaf children must have access to Sign Language. This final chapter has shown that Sign Language is equally indispensable in written language acquisition, which is an integral aspect of the language acquisition process. In our industrialized society, a child's level of interest in the written word is closely linked to how he or she came to value speech and opened up to the world of stories. Thus, the quality of a child's access to speech determines his or her ability to appropriate written language.

For deaf children, *vocal speech* remains an exceptional skill comparable to that of 'the creative artist' (Furth, 1973: 33). On the other hand, *written language* is fully accessible to deaf children, provided they have entered into their full existence as speaking beings through a visual language in which they do not experience any handicap. For them, reading is the door to culture and knowledge.

In deaf education today, 'signs' are recognized to a small degree. Yet their place remains unclear. 'Signs' are allowed as long as they accompany and assist vocal language communication. But this is a far cry from educators truly believing that deaf children must have access to Sign Language. Such a change in attitude is not about to occur soon in French schools.

Although 'signs' are now allowed in deaf education, Sign Language is still almost completely excluded. In terms of communication and language instruction, this is a surprising inconsistency, extremely detrimental to deaf children.

According to Harlan Lane (1980) and François Grosjean (1982), there are two ways of repressing a language. The first is to forbid it, the second, to 'dialectize' it. Dialectization is the form of Sign Language repression currently rampant in deaf education — all under the guise of well-intentioned openness to the world of the deaf! The fact that deaf children are still deprived of the one language fully accessible to them, shows that they are not yet accepted as speaking subjects.

Across the board, schools for the deaf maintain that dialectizing Sign Language ('making it more English-like' (Grosjean, 1982: 87)) helps deaf children understand vocal language syntax. Yet this contradicts linguistic reason. Such an approach frequently leads to misinterpretations of meaning and prevents deaf children from constructing a coherent language system — the very thing upon which a good command of written language depends.

Neither an idol nor a taboo, Sign Language is an invaluable asset in the lives of deaf children — an asset no 'technique' or 'communication system' could ever match. Sign Language allows deaf children to truly understand the structures of language and is thus essential for entering the world of books and literature. This is the process we made possible for the children presented in this book and want to make possible for all deaf children.

In the 1800's, some members of the deaf population were counted among the literary elite of France. It was during this time that Sign Language was recognized and taught in schools for the deaf.

Note to Chapter 8

1. From 'Sophisticated Reading for Children: The Experience of the Classical Jewish Academy' by Leonard R. Mendelsohn in F. Butler, ed., *Children's Literature: The Great Excluded*, Journal of the Modern Language Association Seminar on Children's Literature and the Children's Literature Association, Storrs, Conn.: University of Connecticut, 1973.

Conclusion

Years of working with deaf children as a speech therapist raised many questions in my mind about their speech. To answer these questions, it was necessary to consider the speech process itself and how ordinary children acquire speech.

Part One of this work is the result of that study. An analysis of the nature of the linguistic sign allowed us to depart from an overly instrumentalist view of language. We found that speech is not so much a means of transmitting information as a connecting process. No 'statement' can be interpreted outside the act of its utterance, which is an act of *recognition* between subjects who are talking to each other and whose very existence is linked to the emergence of their own speech. Speech is thus a place where the subject is at once free and constrained. He is free because speech lets him 'become' — prior to speech he does not exist. Yet he is constrained or violated because the act of recognition necessarily forces him to engage in a positioning process with his interlocutor.

In producing speech solely for the pleasure of its sound, the subject escapes the awesome dilemma of speech that simultaneously liberates and oppresses. Playing with signifiers offers each of us a place where we need not distinguish our own speech from that of others. Verbal games are fundamental to the speech process and cannot be relegated to a parallel or secondary phenomenon.

When considered in its full reality, speech loses much of its innocence and transparency. It assumes a flavor and substantiality unacknowledged by theories that view language primarily as a code and as a means for transmitting information.

Once we accept that speech is essentially a 'connecting' process in which subjects come to exist and enter into relationship, we can no longer study it in terms of individual behavior. Speech is comprehensible only within the context of interpersonal relationships. Similarly, only by considering what happens between mother and infant beginning at birth, can we come to understand how infants begin to speak. (Here, 'mother' signifies any person with whom the infant maintains a privileged relationship.)

A mother's first interactions with her infant occur through *multisensory communication* based on eye contact, smiles, touch, cries, vocalizations, mimicry and gestures. Through this *multiplicity of channels*, infants experience their first dialogues.

Well before they begin to talk, infants develop a *competence for communication* that leads to *linguistic competence*. By the time they are six months old, they are able to become *active partners* in ritualized exchanges with their mother. In these exchanges, they master the rules of *turn-taking* and learn *reference* and *predication* techniques that foreshadow verbal communication.

Mothers create an interactive atmosphere that prepares their baby for acquiring speech. In anticipation of their child's communicative abilities, they receive their baby's reactions as *a way of 'telling' them something*, and respond in a perfectly adapted manner that draws their infant into *meaningful dialogue*. Since this response is both verbal and extra-verbal, infants can *understand their mother with their eyes*. In such dialogues, the visual channel is as important as the auditory channel — if not more so. Infants are led to understand the meaning of words through what they *see* in the exchange situation.

Children thus receive their *mother tongue* in an atmosphere of *fun* and *shared pleasure*. Only once a mother *understands* what her infant has expressed in his or her own way will she introduce her baby to the speech spoken by herself and others.

A child's language history begins at birth and is always unique. It is intimately connected to the child's first relationships and the mother's ability to *anticipate* her infant's communicative abilities. This explains why children differ so markedly in their acquisition of language.

It also explains why *all goes well in the opening chapters of deaf children's language history*, provided they enjoy a gratifying relationship with their mother. Vision plays such an enormous role in these first ritualized exchanges between mother and infant that deaf children are not handicapped. They can learn communication skills and develop purely linguistic abilities through pre-verbal dialogue just as other children do. In sum, many more similarities than differences exist in the way deaf and hearing children prepare for speech.

Part Two of this work was devoted to deaf children and the realities of their lives. These observations showed that deaf children of hearing parents begin to suffer increasingly frequent breakdowns in communication beginning at the age of one year. At this age, child-directed speech becomes much less dependent on context, and interactions begin to rely increasingly on the auditory channel. This is also the age at which deafness is often first suspected.

Upon discovering that their child is deaf, hearing mothers often lose their ability to recognize their infant as an active partner in their ritualized exchanges. Once informed that their child cannot hear, they tend to see their infant only in terms of the speech that the child is lacking. They thus become incapable of anticipating their child's verbal abilities and tend to feel speechless themselves. If this breakdown in communication continues, it can cause the child's developing communicative and linguistic abilities to deteriorate instead of blossoming into verbal communication.

On the other hand, preverbal communication develops smoothly in deaf children of deaf parents (in an environment where they are spoken to) and evolves into verbal communication *in Sign Language* at the same age that hearing children begin to speak.

Contrary to widely held beliefs about Sign Language and those who speak it, deaf children are *speaking subjects*. When their parents are also deaf, these children are introduced to the language spoken around them, namely Sign Language, through their *mother tongue*. The fact that the speech these children acquire is visual, does not make it any less real. Through it they come to exist and take on their full stature as speaking subjects.

Deaf children of hearing parents also need to be introduced to the language spoken around them — which they cannot hear. How can a *mother tongue* be restored for these children to bridge the gap between their own way of expressing themselves and the kind of speech used around them? What kind of bridge can connect these two worlds so painfully separated by deafness?

When a hearing mother learns that deaf people have a visual language, her deaf child can once again become an 'infant', that is, a little being received in the *anticipation* that he or she will speak. The mother then realizes that her baby is fully capable of verbal communication provided she uses a visual language. Once she acquires the rudiments of this language, she finds that she can once again speak to her deaf child. By accompanying her vocal speech with signs from Sign Language, she makes her words — which are actually meant to be heard — more clear. This speech modality (called *Signed French* since the signs are produced in French word order) allows a hearing mother to draw her deaf child into speech by adapting her own speech to her child's abilities — which is exactly what all mothers do. She must, however, adapt her speech in a special way. When she does, the processes of speech acquisition are restored: the mother is once again able to anticipate her deaf child's verbal abilities, and an atmosphere of real interaction develops between them. From there, it is not long before she joins other mothers in experiencing the joy of her child's first words — though they be uttered in a gestural modality.

As complete speaking beings, deaf children are destined to become *bilingual*. Once hearing parents understand that Sign Language is the one language that enables deaf children to develop their linguistic abilities without obstacle, they want to let their child learn this language from deaf adults. Thus accepted as different, deaf children come to realize that speaking is also a way of identifying with others. *Vocal speech* then becomes their primary means of satisfying their need to identify with their parents.

Part Three presented a pilot program in bilingual education. The purpose of this presentation, however, was not to prove our theoretical approach. In our view, the *demonstration* of that approach (Part One) stands on its own and in itself establishes the reasons why *Sign Language is a fundamental prerequisite to vocal language acquisition in deaf children.*

The educational philosophy presented here is based on the existence of Sign Language — a poorly understood reality. Yet many people view this philosophy as utopian. Thus, we had to find a way to help make today's 'utopia' become tomorrow's reality.

This is why we presented our pilot program in all its practical aspects, indicating how each related to perspectives defended in our theoretical approach. In this way, we hoped to show how these perspectives could actually become an everyday reality for deaf children, enriching their lives at home, at school and in society.

Sign Language allows deaf children to be received in terms of something *positive*, namely their marvelous ability to express themselves in a visual mode. Their lack of vocal speech is nothing more than the starting point for their education. When deaf children are recognized as linguistic beings and afforded visual speech in a positive atmosphere of communication and accomplishment, they *acquire speech naturally*.

The changes undergone by the children in our class attest to the pleasure they derived from *vocal language* in an educational context where both languages — Sign Language and vocal language — were equally valued. Having discovered for themselves what speaking is about in a language fully accessible to them, they were able to compensate for the gaps they inevitably came up against in vocal language.

Our observations of the children also showed, in a quasi-experimental way, that they acquired words by playing with them, and did so to establish relationships as much as to be able to transmit content. In other words, Sign Language enabled us to establish a teaching environment that respected the necessary conditions of speech acquisition presented in the first, theoretical portion of this book.

In the course of restoring the conditions necessary to healthy language development for these children, we also offered them the opportunity to acquire written language. The development of reading abilities is an integral part of the language acquisition process. The children thus entered into spoken and written language simultaneously.

In depriving deaf children of Sign Language, the hearing world also deprives itself of a richness never imagined in the area of communication and language. When the children in our class were integrated into a hearing school, their language — Sign Language — was recognized and respected. The positive effects that the children and their language had on the entire school revealed what hearing people deny themselves by disregarding Sign Language.

Sign Language could be an excellent means of drawing into verbal communication the inordinate number of kindergartners still uncomfortable with speech. Sign Language can help children who have never experienced multisensory communication regain an appetite for verbal interaction by reawakening in them the visual awareness so essential in the early stages of language development.

Before envisioning the possible benefits of Sign Language to hearing children, however, it is vital to recognize the necessity of this language in the education of *deaf* children. Deaf children must no longer be left without verbal communication during the first crucial years of their lives — as was the case for the six children presented in this book. The moment deafness is diagnosed, parents must be informed that a visual language *does* exist. This would change their whole way of receiving their child. They would perceive their child as an *infant* — a little human being who *will* speak, provided that he or she is spoken to.

As speaking subjects free from obstacle in a visual language, deaf children also become reading and writing subjects, open to all that the world of the written word has to offer.

Appendices

A. Audiometric Curves of the Six Deaf Children in the Bilingual Class

1. Rémi

Right Ear

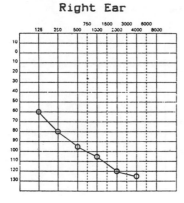

Left Ear

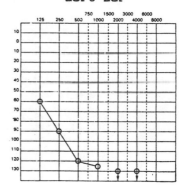

2. Agnes

Right Ear

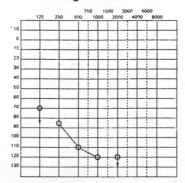

Left Ear

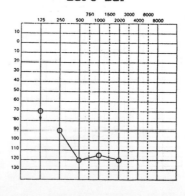

3. Charles

Right Ear

Left Ear

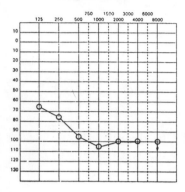
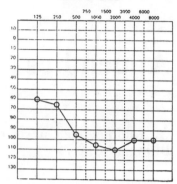

4. Linda
Free Field Exam

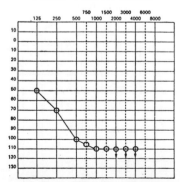

5. Sabine
Free Field Exam

6.Patrick
Free Field Exam

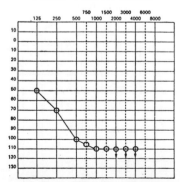
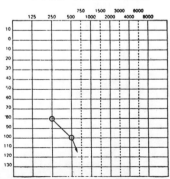

B. The American Manual Alphabet

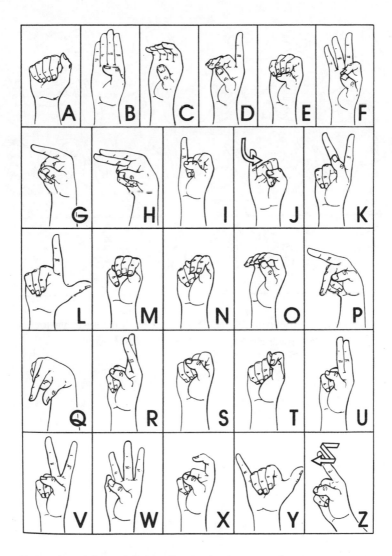

Reproduced from *A Basic Course in American Sign Language* by
Tom Humphries, Carol Padden and Terrance J. O'Rourke
Illustrated by Frank A. Paul with the kind permission of T. J. Publishers Inc.,
817 Silver Spring Ave., 206 Silver Spring, Maryland 20910, USA

C. The Standard British Manual Alphabet

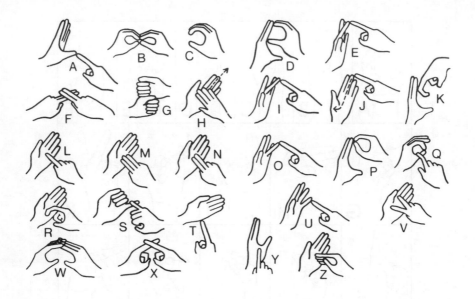

Reproduced with kind permission of The Royal National Institute for the Deaf,
105 Gower Street, London WC1E 6AH, England

References

Ajuriaguerra, J. de. (1972) Désordres psychopathologiques chez l'enfant sourd. *Psychiatrie de l'Enfant* 15(1), 217–244.
— (1974) *Manuel de psychiatrie de l'enfant* (2nd edn). Paris: Masson.
Armengaud, A.-M. and Armengaud, J.-M. (1979) «Itinéraire» d'un enfant sourd. *Rééducation orthophonique* 17(107), 265–274.
Austin, J. L. (1962) *How to Do Things With Words*. Oxford: University Press.
Baker, C. (1976) What's not on the other hand in American Sign Language. *Papers from the 12th Regional Meeting*. Chicago: Chicago Linguistic Society.
Bally, C. (1932) *Linguistique générale et linguistique française*. Paris: Ernest Leroux.
Barthes, R. (1967) *Writing Degree Zero*. Trans. A. Lavers and C. Smith. Boston: Beacon Press. (Originally published (1953) as *Le degrè zéro de l'écriture*. Paris: Editions le Seuil.)
— (1978) Preface to *La parole intermédiaire* by F. Flahault, op. cit.
Battison, R. (1974) Phonological deletion in American Sign Language. *Sign Language Studies* 5, 1–19. Silver Spring: Linstock Press.
— (1978) *Lexical Borrowing in American Sign Language*. Silver Spring: Linstock Press.
Battison, R., Markowicz, H. and Woodward, J. (1975) A good rule of thumb: Variable phonology in American Sign Language. In Shuy and Fasold (eds) *New Ways of Analyzing Variation in English, II*. Washington.
Bellugi, U., Klima, E. and Siple, P. (1975) Remembering in signs. *Cognition* 3, 83–125.
Benveniste, E. (1971) *Problems in General Linguistics*. Trans. M. E. Meek. Corral Gables: University of Miami Press. (Originally published (1966) as *Problèmes de linguistique générale, vol. I*. Paris: Gallimard.)
— (1974) *Problèmes de linguistique générale, vol. II*. Paris: Gallimard.
Berge, F. (1979) Surdité et santé mentale. Témoignage et recherche. *Rééducation orthophonique* 17(107), 241–246.
Best, H. (1943) *Deafness and the Deaf in the United States*. New York: Macmillan.
Bettelheim, B. (1975) *The Uses of Enchantment. The Meaning and Importance of Fairy Tales*. New York: Knopf.
— (1979) The decision to fail. *Surviving and Other Essays*. New York: Knopf.
Bettelheim, B. and Zeland, K. (1982) *On Learning to Read: The Child's Fascination With Meaning*. New York: Knopf.
Bode, L. (1974) Communication of agents, object and indirect object in signed and spoken languages. *Perceptual and Motor Skill* 39, 1151–1158.
Bouvet, D. (1977a) Pédagogie de l'enfant sourd : réflexions à partir de l'oeuvre de M. Degérando. *Rééducation orthophonique*, 15(96), 315–333.
— (1977b) Pédagogie de l'enfant sourd. Compte rendu du Symposium national de Chicago sur la Langue des Signes: Recherche et enseignement. *Rééducation orthophonique* 15(97), 419–441.

— (1978) L'éducation de l'enfant sourd et l'acquisition du langage. *Rééducation ortho-phonique* 16(100), 125–132.
— (1979a) Lettre ouverte aux parents qui ont des enfants sourds. *Handicaps et Inadaptations*. Les Cahiers du Centre technique d'Etudes et de Recherches sur les Handicaps et les Inadaptations, 6 (April–June). 27, quai de la Tournelle, Paris 5e.
— (1979b) De la nécessité de ne pas laisser l'enfant sourd sans communication dès ses premières années. L'apport de la langue des signes. *Audition et Parole vol I*, 4, 151–152.
— (1979c) Le droit de l'enfant sourd à la langue maternelle. *Rééducation ortho-phonique*, 17(107), 225–240.
Brown, K., Hopkins, L. and Hudgins, M. (1967) Causes of childhood deafness. *Proceedings of the International Conference on Oral Education of the Deaf* 77–107. Washington: A. G. Bell Association.
Brown, R. (1977) Introduction to C. E. Snow and C. A. Ferguson (eds) *Talking to Children* op. cit. 1–30.
Bruner, J. S. (1975) From communication to language. A psychological perspective. *Cognition* 3, 255–287.
— (1977) Early social interaction and language acquisition. In H. R. Schaffer (ed), op. cit. 271–289.
— (1978) On prelinguistic prerequisties of speech. In N. Campbell and P. T. Smith, op. cit. 199–214.
Bruner, J. S., Bresson, F. and Piaget, J. (1958) *Logique et perception*. Paris: Presses Universitaires de France.
Bullowa, M. (1979) *Before Speech. The Beginning of Interpersonal Communication.* Cambridge: University Press.
Campbell, N. and Smith, P. T. (1978) Recent Advances in the Psychology of Language: Language Development and Mother–Child Interaction. NATO Conference, Series 4a.
Carroll, L. (1939) Through the looking glass and what Alice found there. In Richard Herick (ed) *The Lewis Carroll Book*. Ill. J. Tenniel and H. Holiday. New York: Tudor Publishing Co.
Clesse, C. (1977) Apprendre à lire en parlant. In L. Lentin *et al.*, op. cit. 91–152.
Collis, G. M. and Schaffer H. R. (1975) Sychronization of visual attention in mother–infant pairs. *Journal of Child Psychology and Psychiatry* 4, 315–320.
Cuxac, C. (1980) Communication visuelle-gestuelle chez les sourds. *Etudes de Linguistique appliquée* 36, 30–40.
Degérando, J.-M. (1827) *De l'éducation des sourds-muets de naissance, vol. I and II.* Paris: Méquignon édit.
Diatkine, R. (1973) Le problème de l'affectivité. *Apprendre à lire: Actes du Symposium sur la lecture*. La Tour-de Pleilz: Ed. Delta, 136–142.
— (1975a) Preface to L. Lentin *Apprendre à parler à l'enfant de moins de 6 ans*, op. cit.
— (1975b) Abord psychiatrique des dysphasies. Paper read to the Association des Rééducateurs de la Parole et du Langage oral et écrit (ARPLOE) on October 24, 1975.
— (1976) Du singulier usage de la parole dans la cure psychanalytique ou de l'intérêt de parler pour ne rien dire. *Revue française de Psychanalyse vol. XL(4)*, 595–604.
— (1980) Communication et langage chez l'enfant sourd. Colloquium in Geneva, November 8, 1980. Service médico-pédagogique.
Diatkine, R., Masse, F. and Mousset, M.-R. (1977) Linguistique et psychopathologie infantile. *Revue de Neuropsychiatrie infantile* 25(2), 117–128.

Dolto, F. (1977) *Lorsque l'enfant paraît*. Paris: Le Seuil.

Doumic-Girard, A. (1980) Développement affectif du petit enfant. *Rééducation ortho-phonique* 18(116),495–508.

Doumic-Girard, A., Male, P. *et al.* (1975) *Psychothérapie du premier âge*. Paris: Presses Universitaires de France.

Ducrot, O. (1972) *Dire et ne pas dire. Principe de sémantique linguistique*. Paris: Hermann.

Ducrot, O. and Todorov, T. (1979) *Encyclopedic Dictionary of the Sciences of Language*. Trans. C. Porter. Baltimore: The Johns Hopkins University Press. (Originally published (1972) as *Dictionnaire encyclopédique des sciences du langage*. Paris: Editions du Seuil.)

Ferguson, C. A. (1977) Baby talk as a simplified register. In C. E. Snow and C. A. Ferguson (eds) op. cit.

Ferreiro, E. (1979) Apprentissage et pratique de la lecture à l'école (communication orale). *Actes du Colloque de Paris, 13–14 juin 1979*. Paris: Centre national de Documentation pédagogique.

Flahault, F. (1978) *La parole intermédiaire*. Paris: Le Seuil.

— (1979) Le fonctionnement de la parole. *Communications* 30, 73–79.

Foucambert, J. (1976) *La manière d'être lecteur*. Paris: OCDL Sermap.

Fraiberg, S. (1974) Blind infants and their mothers: An examination of the sign system. In M. Lewis and L. A. Rosenblum, op. cit. 215–232.

François, F. (1978) *Eléments de linguistique appliquée à l'étude du langage de l'enfant*. Paris: Ed. Baillière, Les Cahiers Baillière.

Freud, S. (1960) *Jokes and their Relation to the Unconscious*. Trans. J. Strachey. New York: W. W. Norton & Co. (Originally published (1912) as *Der Witz und Seine Beziehung Zum Unbewussten* (2nd edn) Leipzig and Vienna: Deutiche.)

Furth, H. (1973) *Deafness and Learning: A Psychological Approach*. Belmont, California: Wadsworth.

Galifret-Granjon, N. (1966) L'apprentissage de la langue écrite et ses troubles. *Bulletin de Psychologie*, XIX(247): 466–474.

Gardiner, A. H. (1932) *The Theory of Speech and Language*. Oxford: Oxford University Press.

Garnica, O. K. (1977) Some prosodic and paralinguistic features of speech to young children. In C. E. Snow and C. A. Ferguson (eds) op. cit. 63–88.

Gelman, R. and Shatz, M. (1977) Appropriate speech adjustments: The operation of conversational constraints on talk to two-year-olds. In M. Lewis and L. A. Rosenblum, op. cit. 27–61.

Gleason, J. Berko (1977) Talking to children: Some notes on feedback. In C. E. Snow and C. A. Ferguson (eds) op. cit. 199–205.

Greenson, R. (1954) About the sound Mm... *The Psychanalytic Quarterly* 23, 234–239.

Grice, H. P. (1975) Logic and conversation. In P. Cole and J. L. Morgan (eds) *Syntax and Semantics, vol. III, Speech Acts* pp. 41–58. New York: Academic Press.

Grosjean, F. (1979) Psycholinguistique et langue des signes. *Langages* 56, 35–57.

— (1982) *Life with Two Languages. An Introduction to Bilingualism*. Cambridge: Harvard University Press.

Guion, J. (1974) *L'institution orthographique*. Paris: Le Centurion.

Halliday, M. A. K. (1979) One child's protolanguage. In M. Bullowa, op. cit. 171–199.

Hammar, A. (1980) The deaf child and the hearing teacher. A bilingual situation. Paper read at the International Congress of Education of the Deaf, August 4–8, 1980, Hambourg.

Hébrard, J. (1977) Rôle du parler dans l'apprentissage de la lecture. In L. Lentin *et al.*, op. cit.

Hess, R. D. and Shipman, V. C. (1965) Early experience and the socialization of cognitive modes in children. *Child Development*, 36, 869–886.

Hockett, C. F. (1958) *A Course in Modern Linguistics.* New York: Macmillan.

Hymes, D. H. (1972) On communicative competence. In J. B. Pride and J. Holmes (eds) *Sociolinguistics* pp. 269–293. Baltimore: Penguin Books.

Jacobs, L. M. (1980) *A Deaf Adult Speaks Out* (2nd edn) Washington: Gallaudet College Press.

Jakobson, R. (1960) Closing statement: Linguistics and poetics. In T. A. Sebeok (ed) *Style and Language.* New York: The Technology Press of MIT and John Wiley & Sons, Inc.

Jesperson, O. (1922) *Language, Its Nature, Development and Origin.* London and New York: Macmillan.

Kannapell, B. (1974) The effects of using stigmatized language. *Deafpride Papers: Perspectives and Options* 9–13.

Kaye, K. (1977) Toward the origin of dialogue. In H. R. Schaffer (ed), op. cit. 89–117.

King-Jordan, I. (1975) A referential communication study of signers and speakers using realistic referents. *Sign Language Studies* 6, 65–103.

Klima, E. and Bellugi, U. (1976) Two faces of sign: Iconic and abstract. *Annals of the New York Academy of Sciences* 280, 514–538.

—— (1979) Iconicity in signs and signing. In E. Klima and U. Bellugi, op. cit. 9–35.

—— (eds) (1979) *The Signs of Language.* Cambridge: Harvard University Press.

Labov, W. (1970) The study of language in its social context. *Studium Generale* 23, 30–87.

Lacan, J. (1973) *Le Séminaire*, liv. I. Paris: Le Seuil.

—— (1977) *Ecrits, A Selection.* Trans. A. Sheridan. New York: W. W. Norton & Co., Inc. (Excerpts from *Ecrits* (1966) Paris: Le Seuil.)

Lane, H. (1980) A chronology of the oppression of Sign Language in France and the United States. In H. Lane and F. Grosjean (eds) *Recent Perspectives on American Sign Language.* Hillsdale, New Jersey: Lawrence Erlbaum Associates.

Leboyer, F. (1976) *Loving Hands.* New York: Knopf.

Lentin, L. (1973) *Comment apprendre à parler à l'enfant: aperçu d'une expérience en cours.* Paris: OCDL, les Editions Sociales Françaises.

—— (1975) *Apprendre à parler à l'enfant de moins de 6 ans.* Paris: Editions Sociales Françaises.

Lentin, L. *et al.* (1977) *Du parler au lire: interaction entre l'adulte et l'enfant.* Paris: Editions Sociales Françaises.

Lepot-Froment, C. (1979) Guidance parentale et développement de la communication chez l'enfant. I: L'instauration du dialogue. *Le Langage et l'Homme* (41).

Leroy, C. (1975) Intonation et syntaxe chez l'enfant français partir de 18 mois. *Cahiers du CREASAS* 13, 33–35.

Lewis, M. and Rosenblum, L. A. (1974) *The Effect of the Infant on Its Care-giver.* New York: Wiley.

—— (1977) *Interaction, Conversation and the Development of Language.* New York: Wiley.

Lieberman, P. (1967) *Intonation, Perception and Language.* Cambridge: MIT Press.

Mackey, W. F. (1976) *Bilingualisme et contact des langues.* Paris: Klincksieck.

Macnamara, J. (1972) Cognitive basis of language learning in infants. *Psychological Review* 79, 1–13.

Maestas y Moores, J. (1979) An ethnographic pilot study of six sets of deaf parents who sign to their infant from birth to 16 months of age. *Proceedings of Recent Developments in Language and Cognition: Sign Language Research*. Copenhagen University.

— (1980) Early linguistic environment. Interactions of deaf parents with their infants. *Sign Language Studies* 26, 1–13.

Maigre-Touchet, A. and Maigre-Touchet, C. (1979a) Lettre à Aurélia. *Coup d'Oeil* 17/18, 12–16.

— (1979b) Aurélia, 4 ans, sourde profonde et la langue des signes française. *Rééducation orthophonique* 17(107), 259–264.

Malmquist, E. (1970) Problems of reading and readers: An international challenge. In D. K. Bracken and E. Malmquist (eds) *Improving Reading Ability Around the World: Proceedings of the Third IRA World Congress on Reading held in Sydney, Australia August 7–9, 1970* pp. 59–71. Newark: International Reading Association.

Malrieu, P. (1979) In Zazzo, op. cit. 106–117.

Martinet, A. (1964) *Elements of General Linguistics*. Transl. E. Palmer. (Originally published (1960) as *Eléments de linguistique générale*. Paris: Librairie Armand Colin.)

— (1968) *La linguistique synchronique*. Paris: Presses Universitaires de France.

McIntire, M. (1974) A modified model for the description of language acquisition in a deaf child. Unpublished Master's Thesis, California State University, Northridge.

— (1977) The acquisition of Sign Language configurations. *Sign Language Studies* 16, 247–266.

McNeill, D. (1970) *The Acquistion of Language*. New York: Harper and Row.

Meadow, K. (1966) The effect of early manual communication and family climate on the deaf child's development. Unpublished doctoral dissertation, University of California, Berkeley.

Meadow, K., Schlesinger, H. and Holstein, C. (1972) The development process in deaf preschool children: Communication competence and socialisation. In Schlesinger and Meadow, op. cit.

Messer, D. J. (1980) The episodic structure of maternal speech to young children. *Journal of Child Language* 7, 29–40.

Meyer, J.-P. and Meyer, L. (1980) Naissance. *Coup d'Oeil* 22, 19–22.

Mindel, E. D. and Vernon, M. C. (1971) *They Grow in Silence*. Silver Spring: National Association of the Deaf.

Montagu, A. (1971) *Touching: The Human Significance of the Skin*, New York: Columbia University Press.

Moody, B. (1979) La communication internationale chez les sourds. *Rééducation orthophonique* 17(107), 213–223.

Moody, B. *et al.* (1986) *Le langage des signes. Entre les mains des sourds, vol. I and II*. Paris: Ed. Ellipses.

Moores, D. (1978) *Educating the Deaf. Psychology, Principles and Practices*. Boston: Houghton Mifflin Company.

Morris, D. (1977) *Manwatching: A Field Guide to Human Behavior*. New York: Harry N. Abrams, Inc.

Mottez, B. and Markowicz, H. (1979) Intégration ou droit à la différence. *Rapport Cordes*. Paris: Centre d'Etude des Mouvements sociaux.

Musset, A. (1844) Pierre et Camille. *Oeuvres complètes en Prose*. Paris: Gallimard (coll. «La Pléiade»), 1960.

Nelson, K. E., Carskaddon, G. and Bonvillian, J. (1973) Syntax acquistion: Impact of experimental variation in adult verbal interaction with the child. *Child Development* 44, 497–504.

Newport, E. L., Gleitman, H. and Gleitman, L. R. (1977) Mother, I'd rather do it myself: Some effects and non-effects of maternal speech style. In C. E. Snow and C. A. Ferguson (eds) op. cit. 109–149.

Newson, J. (1977) An intersubjective approach to the systematic description of mother–infant interaction. In H. R. Schaffer (ed) op. cit. 47–61.

Ninio, A. and Bruner, J. S. (1978) The achievement and antecedents of labeling. *Journal of Child Language* 5, 1–15.

Norden, K. (1980) Learning process and personality development in deaf children, Malmö, Sweden. Paper read at the 3rd International Conference of the European Association of Special Education, August 4–8, 1980 in Finland.

Olèron, P. (1978) *Le langage gestuel des sourds. Syntaxe et communication*. Paris: Ed. du CNRS.

Pagnol, M. (1960) *The Days Were Too Short*. Trans. Rita Barisse. Garden City: Doubleday. (Originally published (1957) as *La gloire de mon Père*. Monaco: Ed. Pastorelly.)

Papoušek, H. and Papoušek, M. (1977) Mothering and the cognitive head-start: Psychobiological considerations. In H. R. Schaffer (ed), op. cit. 63–85, 335, 336, 337.

Pawlby, S. (1977) Imitative interaction. In H. R. Schaffer (ed), op. cit. 203–224.

Pederson, C. (1979) Aspectual modulations on adjectival predicates. In Klima and Bellugi, op. cit. 243–271.

Penfield, W. and Roberts, L. (1959) *Speech and Brain Mechanisms*. Princeton: Princeton University Press.

Perron-Borelli, M. (1976) L'investissement de la signification. *Revue Française de Psychanalyse* XL(4), 681–692.

Pontalis, J.-B. (1975) Trouver, acceuillir, reconnaître l'absent. Preface to D. W. Winnicott *Jeu et réalité. L'espace potentiel*. Paris: Gallimard.

Raynaud, R.-M. (1978) Journées d'information à Monaco. *La Voix du Sourd* (51).

Récanati, F. (1979a) *La transparence et l'énonciation*. Paris: Le Seuil.

— (1979b) Insinuation et sous-entendu. *Communication* 30, 95–105.

Rondal, J. A. (1980) Father's and mother's speech in early language development. *Journal of Child Psychology* 7, 353–369.

Ruesch, J. (1957) *Disturbed Communication*. New York: W. W. Norton.

Saint-Exupéry, A. de. (1946) *Le Petit Prince*. Paris: Gallimard.

Sartre, J.-P. (1964) *The Words*. Trans. B. Frechtman. New York: George Braziller. (Originally published (1964) as *Les mots*. Paris: Gallimard.)

Saussure, F. de. (1986) *A Course in General Linguistics*. Trans. R. Harris. In C. Bally and A. Sechehaye (eds). La Salle: Open Court Publishing Co. (Originally published (1967) as *Cours de linguistique générale*. Paris: Payot.)

Scaife, M. and Bruner, J. S. (1975) The capacity for joint visual attention in the infant. *Nature* 253–265.

Schaffer, H. R. (ed) (1977) *Studies in Mother–Infant Interaction. Proceedings of the Loch Lomond Symposium, September 1975*. Ross Priory, University of Strathclyde. New York: Academic.

Schaffer, H. R., Collis, G. M. and Parsons, G. (1977) Vocal interchange and visual regard in verbal and pre-verbal children. In H. R. Schaffer (ed), op. cit. 291–324.

Schlesinger, H. and Meadow, K. (1972) *Sound and Sign. Childhood Deafness and Mental Health*. Berkeley: University of California Press.

Shatz, M. and Gelman, R. (1977) Beyond syntax: The influence of conversational constraints on speech modification. In C. E. Snow and C. A. Ferguson (eds), op. cit. 189–198.

Siguan e Soler, M. (1977) De la communication gestuelle au langage verbal. In Bronckart *et al. La genèse de la parole. 16 Symposium de Association de Psychologie scientifique de Langue française* pp. 29–68. Paris: Presses Universitaires de France.

Slama-Cazacu, T. (1977) Les échanges verbaux entre les enfants et entre adultes et enfants. In Bronckart *et al. La genèse de la parole. 16 Symposium de Association de Psychologie scientifique de Langue française* pp. 179–240 Paris: Presses Universitaires de France.

Snow, C. E. (1972) Mother's speech to children learning Language. *Child Development* 43, 549–565.

— (1978) The conversational context of language acquistion. In N. Campbell and P. T. Smith, op. cit. 253–269.

Snow, C. E. and Ferguson, C. A. (eds) (1977) *Talking to Children*. Cambridge: Cambridge University Press.

Sperber, D. (1974) *Le symbolique en général*. Paris: Hermann.

Spradley, T. and Spradley, J. (1978) *Deaf Like Me*. New York: Random House.

Stokoe, W. (1978) *Sign Language Structure*. Studies in Linguistics, Occasional Papers, no.8. Buffalo: University of Buffalo, 1960. Reprint, Siver Spring: Linstock Press.

Stokoe, W., Croneberg, C. and Casterline, D. (1976) *A Dictionary of American Sign Language*. Washington: Gallaudet College, 1965. Reprint, Silver Spring: Linstock Press.

Strawson, P. F. (1959) *Individuals: An Essay in Descriptive Metaphysics*. London: Methuen.

Tabouret-Keller, A. (1970) L'acquisition du langage entre deux et trois ans. In M. Cohen *Mélanges*. Paris: Mouton.

Thomas, R. (1979) Un enfant normal. *Coup d'Oeil* 17/18, 11–12.

Vasconcelos, J.-M. de (1970) *My Sweet-Orange Tree*. Transl. E. H. Miller, Jr. New York: Knopf.

Weil, D. (1979) La référence à l'enfant dans quelques travaux de psychologie sur le langage. *Enfance* 3–4 (July–Nov 1979), 293–308.

Weir, R. (1966) Some questions on the child's learning of phonology. In F. Smith and G. A. Miller *The Genisis of Language* pp. 153–168. Cambridge: MIT Press.

— (1970) *Language in the Crib*. The Hague: Mouton.

Wells, G. (1978) What makes for successful language development? In N. Campbell and P. T. Smith, op. cit. 449–469.

Werner, H. and Kaplan, B. (1963) *Symbol Formation*. New York: Wiley.

Wilber, R. and Jones, M. (1974) Some aspects of the bilingual/bimodal acquisition of Sign Language and English by three hearing children of deaf parents. *Papers from the 10th Regional Meeting of the Chicago Linguistic Society*. Ed. Lagaly, Fox and Bruck. Chicago: Chicago Linguistic Society.

Wilson, E. A. (1975) Deafness and mental illness. The rights of deaf patients. Paper read to the Congress of the World Federation of the Deaf, Washington, D.C., August 1975. Repr. in (1976) *Deafpride Papers: Perspective and Option* pp. 25–30. Washington, D. C.

Winnicott, D. W. (1960) The theory of the parent–infant relationship. *International Journal of Psycho-analysis* 40, 585–595.

— (1971) *Playing and Reality*. New York: Tavistok Publications, Ltd., in assoc. with Methuen, Inc.

Wittgenstein, L. (1953) *Philosophical Investigations*. Oxford: Blackwell; New York: Macmillan.

Wyatt, G. (1969) *Language Learning and Communication Disorders in Children*. New York: The Free Press.
Zazzo, R. (1979) *L'attachement*. Paris: Delachaux & Niestlé.

Principal Fairy Tales Cited in Chapter Eight

Little Red Ridinghood
Hansel and Gretel
Goldilocks
Les animaux qui cherchaient l'été
The Nightingale, by H. C. Anderson
The Selfish Giant, by Oscar Wilde